Aspects of selected nursing issues

To the nurses and midwives of Southern Africa

Aspects of selected nursing issues

Charlotte Searle

Butterworths
Durban

© 1988
BUTTERWORTH PUBLISHERS (PTY) LTD
Reg No 70/02642/07

ISBN 0 409 10008 0

THE BUTTERWORTH GROUP

South Africa
BUTTERWORTH PUBLISHERS (PTY) LTD
8 Walter Place   Waterval Park   Mayville   Durban 4091

England
BUTTERWORTH & CO (PUBLISHERS) LTD
London

Australia
BUTTERWORTHS (PTY) LTD
Sydney   Melbourne   Brisbane   Adelaide   Perth

Canada
BUTTERWORTHS CANADA
Toronto   Vancouver

New Zealand
BUTTERWORTHS OF NEW ZEALAND LTD
Wellington   Auckland

Singapore
BUTTERWORTH & CO (ASIA) PTE LTD
Singapore

United States of America
BUTTERWORTH LEGAL PUBLISHERS
Austin   Boston   St Paul   Seattle
D & S PUBLISHERS INC
Clearwater   Florida

Typeset in 10 on 11pt Palitino
by Positone Pinetown
Printed by Interpak Natal Pietermaritzburg

Preface

In the study of the ethos of a profession it becomes necessary to examine the past and the present and to predict the future. What nurses and their leaders say about a specific aspect of the profession at a given time forms the basis for tracing trends in a profession and for speculation about the future.

The addresses collected in this book are all preceded by a short commentary intended to indicate the necessity to review the concepts at regular intervals. It would be meaningful to review the concepts at ten-yearly intervals, for this would demonstrate validity in the thinking and focus attention on the impact of such thinking over a certain period. Over 25 years the impact should be identifiable. This is what the growth of literature and the ethos of nursing and midwifery are all about.

Charlotte Searle
University of South Africa
Pretoria
8 April 1988

Acknowledgements

My special thanks to Sonia van Staden of Butterworths, who expedited proceedings, and Megan Hills, who edited the work. Their wholehearted cooperation is greatly appreciated.

Charlotte Searle

Contents

Part 7 Nursing theories

Part 8 A philosophical perspective

PART

1

General

1

The challenge of a changing world – education, employment conditions, community life

Introductory commentary

This chapter consists of an address given to the Federation of Business and Professional Women. Many nurses are members of this federation and play a leading role in its affairs. Seeing that it is part of an international federation, and that nurses in all parts of the world play an active role in their respective federations, a nurse was asked to present the Corrie van den Bos lecture at the Annual General Meeting of the Federation in 1967.

Corrie van den Bos, a founder member of the Federation in South Africa, was a great educationist, a fighter for women's rights, a friend of the nursing profession and a champion of the working woman. The address forms the background to the contents of this book, which originally saw the light of day as a series of addresses at congresses and discussion groups.

The educational system of a country determines the level of nursing education to which a country can aspire. The nursing system is an integral part of the social system, which is reflected in employment conditions and community life. All professional women share the common heritage outlined in this paper. The facts are relevant to this century and to the beginning of the 21st century. In fact, they are timeless.

THE ADDRESS

Introduction

I am deeply conscious of the honour you have accorded me by asking me to deliver the Corrie van den Bos lecture. I acceded to the request to give the lecture not because I have any profound or original views on the subject under discussion, but because I realise that lectures which have been inaugurated to honour the work of a notable leader and citizen serve to focus the attention of others on the issues with which such a leader concerned him or herself. Thank you for asking me to deliver this lecture. I do so very humbly, for I am only too conscious of the fact that I am speaking to a group of women who are doers in society – persons who invariably play a triple role as professional women or business women and as wives and mothers, each of which is an exacting role and vitally important to the community, economically, socially and culturally.

1

It is a characteristic of organisations such as the South African Federation of Business and Professional Women that they believe implicitly that the strength of a nation depends on the quality of its women. But a credo without action is a poor thing – 'a tinkling cymbal' as St Paul said. In fact, it is merely an ego-booster. Fortunately for the human race in general, and for their own nations in particular, such organisations as yours translate their beliefs into action. Thus they play a critical role in the building of a nation and by their international affiliations make their influence felt in society at large. Therefore I present my thoughts on this subject against the backdrop of your role in society as an organised body of informed, community service orientated women which acts as a pressure group.

Education influences change

Since the subject is a vast one and the real issue in the question of the challenge of change is an educational one, I will endeavour to highlight some of the educational implications that the challenge of a changing world has for employment conditions and community life.

Change we have always had with us. It has been the one great challenge that all living matter has had to face since life first appeared on this earth millions of years ago. Like other living things the human race has shown great resilience and adaptability in meeting the challenges, the buffetings and the pressures of the evolutionary process. It has learned to live with such pressures and to remain master of its fate. Man has now learned to live in outer space, under the sea and on the polar icecaps. Within our lifetime other planets may be populated by emigrants from this planet. Challenge from change there has always been and always will be, so why are we so concerned with the challenge which this technological age is presenting to us? I think our fear is rooted in the fact that the technological revolution has been an extremely rapid one.

We do not know quite how to cope, for we fear that this technological monster, this Frankenstein we have created, will become our master. We realise that developments in the natural sciences and the technological processes resulting from them are making profound changes in our personal and our community life. We fear that scientific and technological progress will overshadow man's finer values. We realise that technology has put untold power within man's reach. We sense that it is threatening man's individuality and that it can lead to his moral destruction. Furthermore, if man does not retain his sense of values then nuclear warfare, the product of this technological age, may well lead to the annihilation of man on earth. Because of the speed with which the technological revolution has overtaken mankind, and because this revolution has shrunk the world to such an extent that we are in fact close neighbours of those living thousands of miles away, it behoves all responsible citizens to take stock of the situation. In doing so we must acknowledge two things, namely that the technological age and its challenges are here to stay, and that we have become involved in the changes brought about by this age without adequate preparation for meeting the challenges emanating therefrom.

'Preparation' is the keywork in accepting challenges. It implies studying the situation, planning, organising and taking action. It implies 'learning' and the 'will' to action.

In other words, the educational process plays a key role in equipping mankind to adapt to change. It gives him the philosophy necessary to face the challenge and provides him with the knowhow to do so. Is this not what man has done since time immemorial?

One has to realise, and of course this is also part of the learning process, that there is nothing to fear in the changes which confront us. With Carlyle (No date 25:352) I say:

> In Change there is nothing terrible, nothing supernatural, on the contrary, it lies at the very essence of our lot and life in this world. Change [is] but the product simply of increased resources which the old methods can no longer administer, of new wealth which the old coffers can no longer contain.

So the answer is simple: find new methods and new coffers.

The learning process has been and always will be the key to man's survival and the survival of those values which set him apart from other living things. It is the tool which makes him master of his fate, for the basis for accepting the challenge in any changing situation is contained in the thoughts so ably expressed by two eminent educationists, Sir JE Adamson (1921:27) and Herman Horne (1927:307), who said respectively: 'education is bringing the individual and the world into relation [with] nature, society and morality' and 'education should be thought of as the process of man's reciprocal adjustment to nature, to his fellows and to the ultimate nature of the cosmos.'

Education is a part of life

Education is not only a necessity *of* life, it is a necessity *for* life in that it is the means of the social and biological continuity of life; in its newest developments even the means of the biological continuity of life from earth to other planets in the universe.

Because education is a necessity for life, the nature of man's adaptation to the challenge of the changes facing him today will depend largely on the type of education he has at his disposal. While accepting the fact that education is a lifelong process (or should be), I am referring particularly to that part of the educational process which is generally regarded as the 'basic educational process' – the time spent at home and at school – for it is this period which lays the foundation for all future endeavour, for further formal or informal education. I regard these two as one, for they should be complementary.

What is taught, *who* teaches it and *how* it is taught are of crucial significance in the educational process. All over the world education is in ferment, because it is realised that these three key factors, *who, what* and *how*, will ultimately determine the quality of man's future. These three elements will be mainly responsible for determining whether in this technological age man will remain master of the machine; whether he will see science and technology as human creations, as tools of the human being, as his servant and not the destroyer of all that which has stood for greatness in the human race.

The most fundamental aspect of the basic educational function is the development of personality and the inculcation of spiritual values and moral principles. It is what I call education for commitment to service, for the preservation of those values which have brought greatness to the human race. It is education for a direction in life and for human growth. Professor WR Niblett (1954:4) has the following to say about this type of educational standpoint:

> I believe that we are not only thoroughly justified in biasing and influencing our children to have standards, to be courageous and believers in truth and freedom, but it is our absolute obligation to do so. Standards, to use the word of JM Cameron, are never simply tame, domesticated belongings, they make claims upon us, preventing us from running uncommitted and unfettered by the weight of humanity's burden we bear.

Education is the basis for meaningful employment and community life

These concepts have meaning for the individual in every walk of life – in the employment situation and in other aspects of community life. They are as basic a necessity as the air that we breathe. The foundation is laid in the home, particularly by the mother, and is further developed at school by teachers in collaboration with parents. The quality of the mothers of our people and of the teachers in our society therefore plays a decisive role in what we are as a nation. As women, and as mothers, the members of an organisation such as yours have a profound interest in those issues which will affect the quality of our homes and of our basic educational institutions. These issues are many and varied, but within the ranks of a multidisciplinary organisation such as yours there are workers who are experts in one or more of the multidimensional aspects of such problems, and your contribution at the national level could be a major one.

Next in importance to this question of personality development and the inculcation of spiritual values and moral principles, indeed part and parcel of it, is the question of human relationships and communication. Fundamental to the art of good human relationships is the art of communication. It is basic to living harmoniously in a changing environment, and harmonious living is a basic requirement for seeing things in their correct perspective and consequently is a requirement for psychosomatic health.

Dr Frances Cloutier, Director-General of the World Federation for Mental Health, said:

> If I were asked what is the most important problem in the world, I would state without a moment's hesitation, that it is the problem of communication between human beings. All other issues, however dramatic they may be, are only different symptoms of our difficulties in understanding ourselves and in understanding others (Cloutier 1969: 1).

The ability to communicate satisfactorily is first acquired in the home environment, where family stability, security and love lay the foundation right from the moment of birth when the mother touches her newborn infant for the first time. The forces which destroy family security weaken a nation immeasurably and have repercussions far beyond the national borders. It is the task of women, in particular, to guard against the violation of the family institution and to lay the foundation for successful communication. At school this is taken a step further. The quality of parents and teachers is decisive in the laying of the right foundations and the creation of a satisfactory climate so that the child may learn the vital art of communicating with his fellow man with circumspection, empathy and clarity. Whether he will be a happy, creative worker, a stable, mature citizen possessing patience and tolerance, will depend on his ability to communicate and on how others communicate with him.

I do not propose to discuss the subject matter of the basic educational course, but I do wish to ask the question whether there should not be a closer approximation between classical and technical education at the basic level. While it is desirable to educate every child according to his abilities and potential, specialisation, whether at the academic or at the technical level, should be delayed as long as possible at school. The essential goals of the basic educational process should be to help the adolescent to live in a technological age as an individual and as a member of a community by imparting to him something of the great cultural heritage of our society, by guiding him to an appreciation of aesthetic and moral standards, by inculcating in him the ability to work efficiently as a member of a group and by providing him with a broad general culture so that he may know how to seize the opportunity to acquire knowledge, to develop his abilities independently and to develop a capacity and a will to analyse problems. To assume responsibility for his personal development he will need to learn how to exercise independent and critical judgement, to balance and to express opinions, to formulate ideas, to exercise initiative, to develop as capacity and a will to work as a member of a team, to adjust swiftly to new working conditions and, above all, to cherish self-respect and respect for others.

Because factual knowledge is so speedily outdated, this approach to the utilisation of individual human resources is essential. The threat that man's individuality will be swamped by technological advances will recede before such a release of human potential.

This type of basic educational preparation acquires greater significance when one realises that the technological revolution is forcing us to look on education as a lifelong process. Continuous evolution in the technological field and increasing automation are, to a greater and greater extent, forcing the world's workers to retrain or to undertake further education at several stages in their working life. If they do not do this they will end up on the labour scrap-heap. This development is also leading to a new type of orientation to the work situation. Because of specialisation and automation workers see only one aspect of the product on which they work. They seldom see the process as a whole. This leads to frustration and job dissatisfaction, and requires greater willpower and concentration from the operator for high quality work. In fact, it is now fairly generally recognised that one of the greatest problems in our economic life, and thus in our social system, is that constituted by those thousands and even millions of workers whose activity can only be described as drudgery because they never have the satisfaction of producing something complete themselves. As a consequence they look upon their work as nothing more than a means of gaining a livelihood. They fail to recognise that the machine is not a dictator, and that to slack in their work means that they will not fulfil their human potential. A new philosophy regarding the role of work in man's life needs to be inculcated to counter such negative aspects. It is in situations such as this that the art of communication, whether up or down the line of authority or horizontally, plays such a major role, for it is in situations such as this that man vents his spite on the machine monster by starting industrial disputes, in which he feels that he is at least pitting his wits against man! It is communication that will make or break man. This is the most fundamental thing we have to learn.

This selfsame technological development is resulting in shorter working hours and more leisure time. Theoretically this is for recuperation purposes, for renewing body and soul so that the treadmill may not appear so oppressive. There is no such thing as leisure time for recuperation purposes if one does not know how to use such time. Education for the enjoyment of leisure time and for the devotion of part of that time to the cause of one's fellow man is imperative. Man does not live in a vacuum, neither can he obtain complete mental and physical well-being if he lives only for himself. Education for social usefulness outside the work and family spheres is also necessary.

Developments in medical science have led to an increase in the life span. If man is to be spared the misery of a lonely and useless old age and the accompanying illhealth which inevitably descends on the lonely or the bored, then education for optimal usage of man's abilities to a ripe old age and for retirement and for social adjustment in old age must begin during the basic education programme so that man can see his life as a whole and can plan accordingly. The qualities which are essential for a happy and useful old age take root during one's early home life and the basic years of schooling. Right from his earliest days man has to be taught that happiness in life and usefulness as a citizen do not depend only on the factual kowledge he acquires about literature, science and the arts, be these the fine arts or the manual arts. All these are indispensable, but he must be made to understand that the development of his personality is paramount, to understand the role he is destined to play in society at large, and to understand that his role must inevitably be blurred if he does not approach his work, his family and his civic duties creatively and with dedication.

To enable their students to meet the challenge of change with regard to employment and community life, the main duty of teachers is to help them to develop independence of thought and the ability to think clearly. An educationist whose name I have unfortunately forgotten once said:

> The real problem which faces educationists is the development of a critical power of analysis, of a capacity to evaluate new ideas, and to stand aside from emotional reactions and to appraise proposals on merit. The scientific attitude of mind is the most urgent necessity to cope with a civilisation cluttered with the product of scientific advances!

I have dealt with the essence of what should be taught in broad outline, and now would like to dwell very briefly on *who* should do this teaching so that man may meet the challenges of the age.

We live in the computer age, when many school children are already learning their lessons in the do-it-yourself manner using automatic teaching machines. Children in the Western world do not find this strange, for they have been brought up on television and a push-button way of life. Teaching machines have a valuable role to play in the teaching of factual subjects, especially in those fields where there is a shortage of teachers, but in a world hungry for education there are too few teachers and the risk that the machine will be used to a greater and greater extent is ever-present. What will the outcome of this be? There is no push-button answer to this question!

As a person who has spent the major part of her life in the professional education field I fear this development, for while there is no denying that these machines have a use in the teaching of factual matter, we have seen that the acquisition of factual knowledge is only one aspect of the educational process and that personality development, communication skill, critical ability and the whole range of qualities discussed previously in fact play the decisive role in the educative process and in man's life. The growth of human values is the answer to the challenge of change, and in this respect the right attitude on the part of the teacher is paramount. Appreciation of human values cannot be acquired by machine learning: it is an attitude of mind that has to be garnered from parents and teachers who themselves have a sound knowledge of all that is best in human values and concerns. In the final analysis the quality of the teacher plays a decisive role. True teachers cherish the relationship which exists between teacher and pupil and cultivate it for the purpose of developing their pupils as individuals who understand the value system of their community. Machines can never replace true teachers. No matter how open-minded we are on this question, we have a duty to ensure that the teaching machine is not used to thin the ranks of teachers for financial reasons. Rather, we should ensure that more and more of our very ablest and enlightened young people are drawn into teaching.

The quality of our educational service is the responsibility of every citizen, and particularly of every woman.

To round off this presentation of ideas on the educational implications of our changing world for employment and community life, I want to highlight a few aspects which concern women in particular, and which should be of special concern to all women's organisations.

The first of these is literacy. Because we are of Africa, children of its soil, we White Africans have a special responsibility to the two hundred million other Africans on this continent to lay the foundations of a dynamic economy which is, after all, the life blood of any nation. We have the wealth and the knowhow to do so. Because we are of Africa we are only too aware that Africa's poverty, her immaturity in terms of 20th century standards, and at times her irresponsibility are rooted in such factors as illiteracy, superstition and a lack of knowledge regarding how to build a modern economy out of the natural resources of the land and the brains, toil and sweat of the people. It has been estimated by UNESCO workers that half of the world's population is illiterate. The percentage of literacy in Africa outside the Republic of South Africa is lamentably low, and efforts to improve this are directed primarily at the male population. Yet here in the Republic we have seen that in Black families it is the mothers who are the driving force in the educational field, and literacy of the mothers has paid handsome social dividends.

The factors which shackle a nation – superstition, poverty, ill-health – have to be tackled at their source, that is in the home, which is the domain of the mother. It is our duty as women to focus attention on this and to help the literacy drives, particularly those directed at the women of Africa. But let us also take a closer look at the education of women in general.

Great demographic changes have characterised the last few decades. In the latter half of the last century approximately 25% of the women in Europe remained single all their lives. Despite the ravages of World War I, only 15% of all girls born in Europe during the first few years of the 20th century remained unmarried, and now an even greater change is facing us. In Britain there are now more young men than women in the age group in which marriage is most likely to occur. The percentage of girls who will not marry is likely to be far lower than it has ever been since statistics have been recorded. Not only will more women marry, but they will do so at a younger age. In Britain one third of all women marry before the age of 21, and it is already estimated that three quarters will be married before they are 25 years of age.

What is the position in South Africa? On 6 September 1960 the population consisted of 8 043 493 males and 7 959 304 females (all races). The mid-year population estimate for 1965 is 8 979 000 males and 8 888 000 females, while the projected population for the year 2000 is 21 159 000 males and 20 814 000 females. If these figures are broken down into the marriage age groups we get the figures in table 1.1.

Table 1.1 Population projection age – male and female as at 30 June 1965 and 2000*

AGE SERIES	WHITE		COLOURED		. ASIATIC	
	1965	2000	1965	2000	1965	2000
15 – 19 years						
Male	163 000	323 000	90 000	307 000	33 000	57 000
Female	156 000	307 000	91 000	305 000	33 000	56 000
20 – 24 years						
Male	143 000	301 000	70 000	252 000	27 000	53 000
Female	138 000	285 000	72 000	249 000	28 000	52 000
25 – 29 years						
Male	124 000	280 000	64 000	208 000	22 000	47 000
Female	120 000	263 000	67 000	206 000	23 000	46 000

* Statistical Year Book 1965, pp A-13 to A-22.
Figures for Blacks were not available.

The young girl of today has a very different life structure from that of her mother. She leaves school at the age of about 16 or 17, works or goes on to further education for about three or four years, and then gets married. She has her children within the first ten years of marriage. She may have to work inbetween having babies and getting them past their infancy, but although she works her primary interest is her home and family. This is, of course, in the national interest. She now has a triple role, that of wife and mother, with the national duty of rearing a stable family, and that of worker, who has a share in turning the economic wheels of the nation. Her burden is immense. Because the nation cannot afford to do without her services as a mother, nor, because of the manpower shortage, without her economic contribution, special consideration should be given to enabling her to fulfil this triple role.

This confronts us with two main educational problems. One concerns the education of women, and the other the education of citizens about the role of women in the modern social structure and about the obligations of society to enable women to fulfil this role. Let us look at the education of women first. We have seen that the prospect of marriage looms on the horizon of every girl. This tends to limit the educational preparation of the majority of women. Many girls and their parents view education as preparation for pre-marriage employment and for employment as an additional source of income after marriage. The result is that many women spend their working lives in jobs in which they cannot realise their full potential because their basic education does not equip them to rise any higher without further study. Far too many of them are not equipped, or prepared, to undertake further study, and do not see education as preparation for a life career.

When a married woman is about 35 or 40 her childbearing years are over, and with the advent of family planning this might well be sooner. Her children are at school all day, or may already be at work. Yet she has some 30 years of active life ahead of her which could be utilised in the labour market. We have to realise, however, that at this stage her work may be totally subordinate to her family interests because her attitudes have been geared by the concept that women's role in the economic field is a temporary or a stopgap one.

Not only does the community need her in the economic field, but it is essential that she is provided with some opportunity to enjoy additional creative experiences in life.

It is time we faced the elementary fact that at some stage or other a married woman will return to work and that without the vast army of workers formed by these women, which amounts to some 33% of the total employed persons in the world, the economy of many nations would be extremely hard hit. But any worthwhile career requires a long period of training, and with earlier marriage becoming the general pattern, fewer girls will enter long training courses. Training for a career before marriage is likely to become even less popular than it has been in the past. We have to acknowledge that for many women training for a career will come, or should come, *during* marriage. Basic education for women should thus be so broadly based that it would be possible to superimpose a career structure on it a considerable time after completion of such basic education.

A burgeoning economy, which is something towards which every nation strives, needs women in industry, in commerce and in the professions to meet the demand for consumer goods and for the services which form the core of a higher standard of living. Therefore thought must be given to creating career structures for married women of mature age. As I have said before, this presupposes a basic educational structure on which a career structure may be imposed, and there lies the rub! We know that married women have come to stay in industry, commerce and the professions. This is the tendency worldwide. Yet their fundamental roles as wives and mothers must not be allowed to suffer. Society, which needs her labour, must therefore make it possible for her to serve in the economic field without sacrificing her major roles. All women need to be educated specifically to make this type of adjustment. Such education should start in early girlhood and continue well into the early years of marriage.

In addition, community education is necessary. Social planners, welfare organisations, employers of labour and voluntary organisations all need advice and guidance on how to assist our growing army of married women workers to carry out their triple role. This is a difficult task. It requires knowledge of the social consequences of neglect of the family institution, knowledge of the extent to which women can carry burdens, and knowledge of the type of social institutions which could be harnessed to help women to fulfil the exacting roles imposed on them by the technical age. Above all, it requires persons of goodwill with a deep sense of social responsibility to initiate and maintain the services which will make it possible for married women to make their contribution to the national economy without jeopardising the social stability of the family, which is the cornerstone of a responsible and stable society.

Women's organisations such as yours have a great responsibility to find the answers to these problems.

Finally, should not we examine the career structure in commerce? Does not this tend to militate against the career woman? With the structure as it exists today, there is very little incentive for girls to pursue lengthy and costly courses which might place them on a rung of the executive ladder in commerce or industry.

In the professions opportunity for advancement is more readily open to women, but we have yet to produce a woman judge in this country.

In conclusion, I want to leave this thought with you. The challenge of a changing world, particularly of this technological age, demands that our social fabric should be constantly strenghtened through our educational process. Commitment to the cause of our fellow man makes all things possible. We can remain the masters of our destiny only if this process is hammered out under the searchlight of science on the anvil of integrity, faith, hope, love and charity!

References

Adamson, Sir JE. 1921. *The Individual and the Environment*. Longman Green.
Carlyle, T. (No date). Characteristics. *Howard Classics* 25: 352.
Cloutier, F. 1969. *Address*. World Federation of Mental Health, Geneva.
Horne, HH. 1927. *The Philosophy of Education*. New York: Macmillan.
Niblett, Prof JR. 1954. *Education, Bias and Indoctrination*. University of Leeds Institute of Education. No 9 Researches and Studies.

PART 2

The role of the nurse administrator
– what is it? (an ethos perspective)

2

The role of the matron (nurse administrator)

in the modern hospital

[A 1951 South African perspective]

Introductory commentary

In 1951 the Transvaal Provincial Administration introduced a course for nurse administrators. The aim was to revitalise and modernise nursing service in the provincial hospitals. The course led to a Diploma in Nursing Administration (Hospital and Health Services) and was of an experimental nature. Five years later the SA Nursing Council registered the diploma as an additional qualification in nursing. Many years later the Council promulgated regulations for a Diploma in Nursing Administration and became the examining body. The experimental course became a Nursing Council course.

At that time the concept of the role of the matron was based on that applicable in Great Britain. Gradually a typically South African slant was given to the course to meet the specific needs of the health care system in this country.

The course has had an immense effect on the development of the nursing services in South Africa. Today it is a compulsory requirement for promotion to the upper echelons of the nursing service.

Concepts have been modified over the years. Except in small hospitals, the domestic service is no longer the concern of the matron. She is no longer the mother of the house or the mistress of the household! Or is she? Being part of the top management structure of a health service gives her a particular strength as mistress of the household. The power she can wield, the responsibilities that are encompassed in this concept govern the entire range of her service. She is the boss of it all. Why has she retreated from this position of strength?

Examine this chapter. See whether it contains certain fundamental truths which must be carried forward into the future. Every modern function the matron has to perform can be slotted into the concepts that formed the basis for the development of the academic and functional activities encompassed by the concept nursing administration. The present decade is adding the trimmings to these concepts. Teaching and organisational approaches are being modernised, but the essential truths live one!

Note: The terms 'nurse administrator' and 'nurse manager' are used interchangeably.

THE ADDRESS

Ever since temples and houses of healing were founded, a Chief Temple Woman or Priestess or Mother of the House has occupied a key position in the organisation. Her function was simply that of mistress of the household. A mother in a home occupies a unique position in the life of the family. Her whole life is devoted to but one purpose, namely the welfare and happiness of her family. She creates a happy home for its members, operates her household budget frugally, educates her children wisely, directs her household workers justly and deals with the fears and grief of her family and household at all times. She is the cornerstone on which the security of the household rests.

Down the centuries the work of healing has been passed on and has multiplied as a result of the selfless and untiring devotion of women who organised the services for the sick and acted as mothers of the houses for the sick. They tended, comforted and educated mankind, organised great services to make their work of mercy more effective, and, in so doing, passed on an immortal heritage of service and knowledge to the generations which were to follow them. These women laid the foundations of modern hospital work, for not only did they make hospital work an art, but the skill of the physician and surgeon rose to the great heights it has reached today by virtue of the organisation of hospitals and the training of skilled nurses who provided the correct field for the medical practitioner to practice his art.

The modern counterpart of the Chief Temple Woman or Mother of the House is the Matron or Chief Nurse Administrator in a hospital or nursing service. In fact, in the Transvaal Provincial Nursing Service, the term 'matron' is defined as the 'mistress of the household'.

Let us look at the modern 'mistress of the household'. What are her functions and what is the ethical concept which her post, her actions and her being should typify?

The matron acts as coordinator-in-chief of the members of her own team, but also functions in this capacity for the health team as a whole, for all services which reach a patient do so either directly or indirectly through the nursing service. It is self-evident, therefore, that her main function is the organisation and management of the physical facilities and personnel resources necessary for adequate patient care. The purpose of her existence is to provide these in order to keep her fellow citizens in good health or to restore them to good health and while doing so to bring peace and happiness to them all. She is managing a professional service to the sick. This is the essence of her task.

Humanity is seething with unrest and frustration which is resulting in mental and physical breakdown in very large numbers of people. Therefore good organisation and management of health services is a matter of supreme importance to national survival. The matron plays a leading role in the organisation and management of such services. She is the chief coordinator of the health team. In this position, in which she is responsible for the organisation and management of things as well as of human services, she needs extensive knowledge of the fundamental principles of organisation and management.

She must possess detailed knowledge of the service which she controls and, in addition, must have a very clear concept of the function and manner of organisation and management of all other services which impinge on her specific field of service. Above all, she must have a very clear idea of the purpose of the organisation as a whole, the methods to be employed to reach the desired objectives and the countermeasures which may be applied when breakdowns threaten.

Her function is that of an organiser. In *Organize* Herbert Casson (No date:37-42) states:

> . . . the greater part of the work of an Organiser can be summed up in three words – learning, thinking and planning . . . the difference between a worker and an Organiser is that the worker aims at DOING whilst an Organiser aims at GETTING things DONE.

This is the crux of the matter. Managing is essentially different from working. There is a definite limit to what can be done by one human being, but there is practically no limit to what a good organiser can do through the efforts of others.

It has been said that many matrons run around in circles. Why is this so? Fundamentally it is due to the fact that they have a sound knowledge of nursing, but little knowledge of administration. They have not learned to give their attention to planning, organisation and development. They have not learned to delegate some of their duties to competent lieutenants.

An analysis of the functions of a matron in a modern hospital organisation indicates that there are a great many facets of hospital service which she must integrate into one purposeful whole in order that the single objective of hospital activity, namely good patient care, may be achieved. In order that this may be achieved certain major responsibilities are placed on her. Enumeration of these responsibilities should serve to outline the scope of the post she holds. In modern hospitals the matron is the head of the nursing and domestic services. As such she is responsible to the Medical Superintendent (or the Board of Governors if there is no Medical Superintendent) for:

(i) the organisation of the physical conditions for adequate nursing care in any type of clinical service where nursing service is rendered in any form

(ii) the provision of quality nursing care to any type of clinical condition that may be present in the hospital or those admitted to it

(iii) the organisation and maintenance of a nursing and domestic force which will be able to cope satisfactorily with the demands made on them by the clinical and domestic services, bearing in mind that at all times quality is to be the keynote in this type of organisation

(iv) the acts and omissions of service personnel whom she directs

(v) the installation of approved systems of expense control within the services which she directs and the administration of all her departments on sound business lines, that is maximum efficiency is to be obtained on minimum costs

(vi) the integration of ancillary services with her departments without friction and wasteful expenditure. Smooth-flowing interdepartmental activity in an organisation as complex as a hospital service is essential, otherwise every task would constitute a major emergency. The diplomatic action which mades this possible is of the greatest importance in hospital organisation

(vii) the provision of appropriate education for all the personnel under her command

(viii) the management of all personnel issues which fall under her jurisdiction, including the health protection and welfare of such personnel

(ix) the control of medical hazards in as far as this is possible within the area of her control.

If a matron is to carry out these duties efficiently it is necessary that she has a very clear concept of the functional activities of such services and knows exactly what her personnel resources are and how these may best be used to give maximum production with minimum effort.

In order that her organisation of the physical conditions for nursing care may be effective it is necessary that she is a member of the team which plans the development of the various clinical services and the services ancillary thereto, and she should see to it that there is an economical grouping of the components of the various ward units so that finishes, fitments and equipment are suitable and adequate for maximum efficiency. This implies that she should have made a comprehensive study of functional planning, organisation and the commissioning of services and acquisition of hospital equipment.

In order that she may organise and maintain an adequate nursing and domestic force, it is necessary that she has a thorough understanding of the functions, management and scope of the services to be rendered by these groups. An analysis of the activity fields of these groups would indicate what type of worker should be used, the extent of the services to be rendered by each grade of personnel and the educational programme necessary to prepare workers for the various fields. Job analysis and educational direction thus form part of her manifold duties.

It is quite impossible for any head to attend to all the activities of a complex organisation such as a hospital. Therefore it is necessary that the matron delegates some of her authority. To her many duties is added one of the most vital duties of all, that of Chief Personnel Manager. If necessary she has to dip deep into the staff bucket to bring able officers to her assistance. She must forget her dislike of delegating some of her responsibilities or imparting any of her knowledge. Her chief function is to lay down policy, create a competent assistant force to carry it out, and supervise and assess the process. Her measure of success and her influence on posterity will be gauged by the power she leaves behind her. Therefore it is imperative that as a nursing service grows the principal matron spends time on the search for and development of dependable assistants and workers, and on passing knowledge down the line.

The fundamental principles of good management are thinking, studying, planning, teaching, supervision and the assessment of the end product of functions. Therefore the penultimate job of the chief matron is to study the service that she is organising and, above all, the human beings who carry out this service, in order that she may create a well-functioning service. She must study every facet of it, devise an appropriate routine (by experimentation if necessary), and, when a humane and economical routine has been devised, must leave it alone and concentrate on the human beings who are going to do the job. To find the right person for every job requires careful study and a great deal of teaching. Not only should she direct or provide for the teaching of technical skills, but she should teach the ethical basis of the work to all her workers by precept and example. In other words, she must be the team leader. She must respect her workers, their authority and status, and in so doing she will ensure that they, in turn, respect their fellow workers, so that inter-personnel and interdepartmental harmony results. She must hold the reins confidently and expertly and drive the chariot to its destination. She must not attempt to be the horse which pulls the chariot!

It has already been said that the direction of education is one of the major responsibilities of the matron. At present this includes training domestic workers of all grades and educating and training nursing personnel at the basic as well as the post-basic level. It is in this area that the greatest test of the quality of a matron's leadership is made. She constantly has to reconcile the conflicting needs of the educational programme and the service. It is her responsibility to strike a balance between the two. She must acquaint herself thoroughly with the principles underlying the various educational programmes, as she cannot direct these unless she has detailed knowledge of their functional purpose. It is her duty to provide the facilities for and direction of such programmes with regard to the social as well as professional aspects. Deep understanding of the principles involved is basic to it all, for moulding the lives of other people is a very grave responsibility.

Serving the immediate needs of the hospital is not enough. The organisation must provide for future as well as present needs. Hospital service is a continuous service which must keep abreast of the times. Nursing organisation and nursing education is crucial in this respect. A matron's responsibility in the educational field is therefore most important.

The matron's responsibilities do not end with the organisation she serves. She also has to make her weight felt in the community. Social, educational and economic dislocation in the community causes breakdowns in health. It is the duty of the matron, as of every health worker, to make her wealth of knowledge and experience available to the community she serves. Therefore she should not live in cloistered seclusion, but should take part in community activities which endeavour to combat social dislocation.

The main roles of a matron are the management of services and the education of personnel and she must have many vital qualities to fulfil her roles satisfactorily. She must have good judgement, firmness, alertness, fairness, the ability to select staff, teaching ability, likeableness, courage, stamina, wisdom, patience and, above all, a great love for and faith in the work she is doing. No person can lead well unless she has complete faith in what she is doing and an all-consuming love for the cause.

A matron must be able to inspire those who work with her. She must be able to make each work unit, no matter how humble, feel that he/she has a really important contribution to make and that his/her effort is appreciated.

A matron's greatest role lies in presenting the organisation to her staff and allied personnel as a dynamic organism which thrives on love, faith and honest service, gladly given.

It will be necessary to review this standpoint every five years. This will be your task. You will be able to do so effectively only if you fully understand the content of the course you have embarked upon. Be guided by what Casson (II no date:18) stated:

> Man succeeds by the number and wisdom of his creative actions. His never-ending task is to act wisely.

References

Casson, HN. (I) No date. *Organize*. London: The Efficiency Magazine Publishers.
Casson, HN. (II) No date. *How to get things done*. London: The Efficiency Magazine Publishers.

3

The nurse administrator as a pioneer of health

[A 1954 international perspective]

Introductory commentary

Nursing administration has been with mankind since the first Temples of Healing of early Greek civilisation and the Houses for the Sick of early Indian civilisation. The description in the *Charaka Samhita* (one of the compendiums of the holy books of India – the *Ayur Veda*) of the organisation and management of the Houses of the Sick indicate that there must have been a type of nursing service manpower.

Similarly, the Greek Temples of Healing required some form of administration of the facilities and the nursing care provided by the temple maidens. Therefore, nursing administration has its roots in the distant origins of man's life on earth.

The address below was given at a seminar to commemorate the centenary of the work of Florence Nightingale in the Crimea. The thoughts expressed are timeless; they serve as a link between the past and the future in nursing administration. The philosophy that permeates the address is that which underpins nursing administration now, three decades later. The address has meaning for the contemporary professional nurse: it demonstrates the continuity of the thread of nursing administration in the development of health care and the lasting truth of the philosophy which forms its foundation.

The address is in reality a message to the nursing profession that, despite the onslaught by other categories of administrative personnel on the concept of nursing administration, the nursing profession must stand firm and retain that which is its own. It must forge strong links between the past and the future, for the ethos of nursing in this country will be profoundly affected by the quality of nursing administration and whether this remains in the hands of the nursing profession. Florence Nightingale is the prototype of the modern nurse administrator. How the profession entrenches its right to administer the nursing services will show how nurses in the latter quarter of the 20th century have kept faith in Florence Nightingale's precepts, vision and ideals.

THE ADDRESS

Down the centuries of man's existence a light has burned steadily. Sometimes it has burned but dimly, while at others it has blazed fiercely. It has its source in the continuous and selfless devotion of thousands of men and women who have dedicated their lives, their love and their talents to the care of their fellow men. The long, glorious and oft-times troubled history of the nursing profession is apt to fade into the shadows of the past, but today we humbly remember that 100 years ago a brave, compassionate woman left the shores of Great Britain for the Crimean battle field with a small band of helpers. All the civilised world knows the immortal story of Florence Nightingale and her band of nurses who braved the horrors, the filth and the degradation of Scutari, and in so doing set a pattern for modern nursing which has reached the farthest corners of the earth. We remember her and her deeds and we humbly thank God that in His wisdom He sent Miss Nightingale to organise the prototype of this greatest of all modern humanitarian services, the nursing service.

But we should also remember and return thanks that the flame which burned so brightly in the heart of Florence Nightingale has always been with mankind, and that there have been great men and women who nurtured this flame and passed it along to the next generation. We find the story of these men and women in the chronicles of the ancient races which existed long before the birth of Christ. We find their names in pagan as well as Christian communities.

They were the people whose lives so influenced a wealthy, high-born lady that she joined hands with them over the centuries and carried on what they had begun. Today we honour Miss Nightingale, modern nurse and nurse administrator without equal, but we also remember, among others, Phoebe of Cenchrea, the friend of St Paul, who organised the first known District Nursing Service; Paula, the wealthy Roman matron who organised the first Christian hospital; Queen Elizabeth of Hungary, who combined nursing and social welfare work; and Pastor and Frau Fliedner, who organised modern hospital and welfare work and influenced the wealthy Miss Nightingale so profoundly.

Why have these names been handed on as part of our sacred heritage as nurses? The sublime love and compassion of these people, their ceaseless sacrifice and the nobility of their lives were dominated by their great ability to organise and by their desire to pass their skill and knowledge on to the next generation. They all organised great services which left a lasting mark on mankind. They were great nurse administrators. The men and women they influenced went far afield and carried their message of devoted service to all corners of the earth. Their message of faith, hope and charity has spanned the world.

Only a few years after Florence Nightingale started the first training system for professional nurses one of its first products arrived in South Africa. She was Sister Henrietta of the Order of St Michael and All Angels. A devout Christian, devoted nurse and great administrator, she is remembered in South Africa and the British nursing world as the woman who pioneered promotive health nursing, modern midwifery and institutional nursing in South Africa. She was tireless in her efforts to bring health to the people of South Africa.

Not content merely to organise nursing services and hospital facilities, Sister Henrietta also pioneered South African nursing and midwifery education and started the first nursing schools. She also campaigned ceaselessly for state recognition of these professions and in 1891 succeeded in securing state registration for these professional groups before it existed in any other country in the world. Like the nurses of old, she made sure that she handed on not only a great example of devotion of skill, but wide knowledge of administrative skills.

The South African professional nursing service was born on the diamond fields of Kimberley amidst squalor, sickness and undreamed of degradation on the one hand, and fabulous wealth on the other. Within a matter of 10 years the products of Sister Henrietta's training system were to be found in all parts of South Africa and even in the Rhodesias. The honoured position held by nurses in South African to this day and the high ethical standard expected of them dates back to the Henrietta period in South African nursing history. She was an administrator whose work will live on in Southern Africa for as long as civilisation continues here.

It is now World Health Day, 1954, and we are commemorating the work of Florence Nightingale in the Crimea. The World Health Organisation has set as the theme for this commemoration 'The Nurse Pioneer of Health'. Small wonder that my thoughts have turned to Sister Henrietta, the nurse administrator who pioneered health in South Africa. From her work we see that her greatest contribution lay not only in tending the sick herself, but in organising a nursing service. This was the pattern set by Florence Nightingale. Her purpose in nurse training was a dual one. She aimed at producing bedside nurses who had sufficient skill and initiative to organise nursing services so that their own knowledge could be spread as far afield as possible. Today we find that nurses are well in the vanguard of the crusade for improved health conditions that the World Health Organisation is conducting in so many parts of the world. What is the chief function of these World Health Organisation nurses, and what is the chief function of nurse administrators all over the world? They are all people who are technically thoroughly proficient, but their chief service is to prepare the conditions in which other members of the health team exercise their calling. They go into the field as organisers and administrators. The function of the nurse administrator is best described by Herman Finer (1951:4) in 'Administration and the Nursing Services', in which he states:

> Nursing Administration is the system of activities directed toward the nursing care of patients, and includes the establishment of overall goals and policies within the aims of the health agency and provision for organisation, personnel, and facilities to accomplish these goals in the most effective and economical manner through co-operative efforts of all members of staff, co-ordinating the service with other departments of this situation.

We need to study this process of nursing administration. Urwick (1951:10-11) says:

> [the] modern concept of management – the business term for administration – must be learned . . . in the art of administration we are as yet barely adolescent.

From this we can see that the nurse administrator holds a key position in any health field, be it hospital, public health or district nursing team. It is she who coordinates the activities of her group into a purposeful whole. Not only does this coordination extend to members of her own team, but she acts as the chief coordinator of the health team as a whole, for all services which reach a patient do so either directly or indirectly through the nurse. Those nurses who take on administrative duties assume a responsibility which never ends, for they must not only serve the present generation, but also build to provide for a continuation and extension of the service when they are no longer there. This is the most vital and sacred trust which is imposed on them. Not through them must the flame be dimmed or die down. They must constantly add to the fuel in the lamp so that it may reach the next relay of nurse administrators, burning brightly.

Today nursing administration centres around the concept that nursing embraces the whole patient, physically and mentally, and endeavours to adjust the patient as a whole being to his environment. Today's nurse accepts that the provision of a suitable environment is as much her concern as the care of the patient. Nursing administration which subscribes to these ideals must have the vision to centre its nursing care on the group concept, with a strong individual-centred care performance. The level of the detailed individual attention will be determined by the strength of the ethical code to which the nurse administrator and her nurses subscribe.

Nurse administrators in South Africa have long been pressing for more adequate preparation of nurses in the social and psychological fields, for they have realised that the reactions and mechanics of human behaviour are inseparable from the fields of physical and mental health. The South African nursing service is making a determined effort to equip every nursing unit with basic knowledge in these fields, and we hope that other allied health professions in South Africa will follow this lead.

Seeing that nursing administration involves the organisation of physical facilities as well as human resources, and that a nurse administrator must have a thorough knowledge of how to analyse community requirements and service needs, it has long been felt that the greatest tribute that could be paid to the work of Miss Nightingale would be to prepare nurses in such a way that they could administer nursing services. The long and arduous basic training course in South Africa does not qualify nurses for administrative duties beyond those of a sister. Administrative skill is usually acquired over years of experience. It has been recognised, however, that practical experience may be of such a nature that a 'one-track' mind results. To improve the situation and to meet the growing demands of the hospital services in South Africa, in 1951 a course for nurse administrators was devised. The purpose of this course is not to supply the nurse with a bag of administrative tricks, but to teach her the principles which underlie administration in general, and hospital administration in particular. The fundamental purpose of the course is to give her a sound grounding in the social sciences and the principles of nursing education, both basic and advanced, as well as in the principles which are fundamental to the organisation of the physical and human resources of the hospital. A determined effort is made to develop judgement. There is no place in the modern nursing world for a person who administers a service by means of a fixed set of regulations. It is impossible to prescribe regulations for all the situations which may arise in the nursing service.

The nurse administrator is taught to use regulations wisely, to analyse situations as they arise and to endeavour to find a workable and just solution to problems. Needless to say, all who offer themselves for such courses are not 'Henriettas'. Nevertheless, they will extract all they can from the accumulated wisdom of the past, build on it, and use their talents wisely for the pioneering of health in their community. They will be the ones who will reach across the years to come and pass on the heritage of service to mankind and good health to every citizen.

References

Finer, H. 1951. *Administration and the nursing service*. London: ICN. (Draft copy).
Urwick, L. 1951. *The elements of administration*. London: Isaac Pitman & Sons.

The training of nurses for management

[A 1973 international perspective]

Introductory commentary

There is a need to develop a standpoint regarding the education and training of nurses for management. This must be such that it will allow this particular educational process to extend well into the future. All concepts must be able to stand the test of time, in whichever country they are applied. The fact that a nurse's management training should begin during the first year of her basic preparation is frequently overlooked, as is the fact that management training should form part of the entire period of professional practice. Management training in nursing spans the professional life of a nurse from when she enters nursing school to when she is doing her doctoral preparation at university.

The concepts which received international acclaim at an international Hospital Federation Congress have meaning for the survival of the role of nurse administrator.

The concepts enunciated are aimed at developing a specific ethos of nursing administration.

THE ADDRESS

Some 2000 years ago Cicero proclaimed that 'confidence is that feeling by which the mind embarks on great and honourable courses with a sure hope and trust in itself'.

The ultimate purpose

Education for management in all its aspects, in all its diversity, has the development of such confidence as its ultimate objective, irrespective of the field in which such management preparation is undertaken.

In any undertaking, success depends on the quality of management. Management is a preoccupation with the age-old problem of the multiplicity of ends and the scarcity of means.

The consequences of expanding services

Within the nursing profession confident management expertise is inadequate to maintain existing nursing services satisfactorily. Future health service needs will aggravate the problem a thousandfold.

Nursing is the pivot about which the entire health service revolves. Therefore nursing management has a critical role to play in the provision of health services and it will have to play this role in a milieu in which competition for available resources is increasingly keen.

Nursing management has to recognise that nursing has to contend with not only a scientific revolution in medicine, but also a social revolution in the community, to the extent that it is now generally accepted that changing conditions require the reorientation and retraining of personnel in management methods and attitudes at least three times during a working life span. This applies to the professional worker as much as it does to the worker in industry.

Nursing must recognise this at a time when it is failing to meet existing needs, even though (in most Western countries at least) there are far more qualified nurses available than the health services can absorb. Many qualified nurses who would be employed in the health services are gainfully employed in other fields or are not working at all because contemporary methods of organisation and management in nursing services actually prevent their employment as nurses. The lack of effective organisation and management and traditionalism has created a situation amounting to famine amid plenty. Not only nurses, but also administrators, doctors and politicians are responsible for this. The wastage of nursing resources will increase unless top management in the health services, medical, nursing and general, combine to seek a remedy. It is obviously not only a matter of urgency, but one calling for the sustained application of high level managerial skill.

It is equally obvious that such managerial skill can come only from personnel whose attitudes and abilities are such that they are able to move with the times, are able to analyse needs and trends, have the knowledge and confidence to plan and implement new ways of doing things, and have levels of competence and expertise which demand respect for their views from higher authorities. This is possible only if the authorities find that the proponents of change not only have the welfare of the organisation and of the personnel at heart, but are also versed in the ways of attaining defined objectives and have achieved that acme of executive ability, namely the ability to convert knowledge, skill and vision into effectiveness. This is the only type of management language that has any meaning whatsoever.

Nurses and health planners have to take note of the fact that at the beginning of this century seven out of ten workers in the great industrial countries were directly involved in the production of goods. It is estimated that by 1980 this figure will have dropped to three, because machines will be the great producers of goods. The other workers will be employed in ultrasophisticated service industries. From cradle to grave, as they progress and as they become urbanised, people want more and more things done for them. Already there appears to be a tendency to relate national status less to the gross national product and more to the extent and level of sophistication of the services that a nation renders its citizens and other countries in less affluent circumstances. So extensive have many service industries become that they require other service industries to keep them going, and this is the case with nursing.

A service orientated economy must inevitably draw larger and larger numbers of women into gainful employment outside their homes. This, in turn, will create a service industry relating to the care of infants, toddlers and pre-school children which will compete strongly with the health service industry for personnel. In 1976 the estimated number of hospital beds in the USA was 1 927 000. In the same period the estimated number of toddlers and pre-school children of some 5,3 million working mothers was 8 000 000. Moreover, there were millions of children of primary school age who needed after-school care to avoid 'latch key' problems in early childhood.

The service needs of these two vulnerable groups, children and those in need of health care, compete with each other for scarce personnel, although these services should be complementary. And so the picture can be expanded. The common denominators in the expansion of health and other service industries are a shortage of personnel and material resources and an excess of aspiration for further expansion. Therefore we must make the most of what we have or are likely to have.

In the health services, where the overwhelming proportion of service must be given on a 24-hour basis 365 days a year, the impact of the expansion of service industries in which women are employed is particularly heavy. Meanwhile, the millstone of outmoded concepts of nursing management threatens to drag our services under water.

The population explosion, the trend towards earlier marriage among young women, the rise in the population age level in most nations, changes in ways of life and family patterns which reduce family participation in the provision of health care, the disproportionate development of expensive institutional health services at the cost of basic preventive and promotive health services, and the tradition-bound practices of doctors and nurses all aggravate our difficulties. Add to this a level of economic affluence which enables workers to shun demanding, high-risk jobs with unpopular working hours, and it can be seen that top management in the health services has a very difficult furrow to plough. The quality of management will have to be higher than it has ever been if nursing services are to be maintained under such demanding and highly competitive conditions, where the annual growth rate of the services far exceeds the annual growth of the population.

Clearly, education for nursing management is necessary if we are to meet health needs at even a maintenance level.

Management education generally

The function of management is essentially to get things done. It is action – the development of human and material resources to obtain an optimal level of production with minimal expenditure and utilisation of scarce resources. Successful management is an accomplishment requiring study, knowledge, skill, foresight, experience, courage and the confidence to make well-timed, effective judgements and not rule-of-thumb decisions. It is a way of life, not something which can be grafted onto a person once he or she is already well settled in his or her chosen career. It is the product of growth which has its roots in the basic education for a career to which the individual has been exposed and in the role he has played so far in his productive life. Thereafter specific management education, whether ad hoc, diploma or degree courses, adds the essential polish. It is important that high level management courses should be taken at an age when the individual has learnt to assess with discrimination what has to be learnt and is able to do so, at an age where the fires of enthusiasm are still burning and before the iron bands of tradition have imprisoned the individual. I see the process as a continuing one comprising four phases:

(i) basic professional education
(ii) continuing as well as in-service education
(iii) advanced education
(iv) lifelong non-formal continuing education.

Management education for nurses

As important as formal courses in management theory are, so too is the concept of continuous education for management. Educating nurses for management should be a continuous process which begins when they enter nursing school and continues until they retire as senior nursing executives. In educating nurses for management it is our duty to ensure that all along the line the personal potential and attitudes of nurses are given maximum opportunity to grow and mature. This includes attitude potential and management potential. Attitudes either block or liberate management potential.

The foundation for top management in nursing must be laid during the basic nursing course. This is where education for nursing management must start. Some nursing educationists and health authorities do not agree with this and organise basic nursing courses in such a manner that management potential is either discouraged or stultified. As a result subsequent efforts to graft on this vital functional ability in later years are not always very successful.

There are actually two opposing schools of thought in basic nursing education whose philosophies regarding management education at the basic level ultimately have a negative result. On the one hand there is the school of thought which is so philosophical about nursing education that it loses sight of reality. This school stresses the study of the science of nursing and its supportive sciences, and cuts clinical experience to a bare minimum. The idea that the student should actually form part of the working team in the health service situation, that she should gain experience not only in the care of individual patients, but in the handling of the total system of providing care to a group of patients for whose welfare she personally has to account, is rejected. Service is a dirty word. This, proponents of this school say, is not part of nursing education. Their view denies the student sufficient opportunity to learn by doing and the opportunity to test fully in the practical situation what she has learnt in the classroom. The student cannot learn how to cope with the health needs of groups of people unless she is a full member of a clinical team for a substantial portion of her basic professional preparation. She may become an expert in individual patient care, but while this is laudable in itself it is not enough, because the diversity and complexity of mass patient needs elude her.

Millions of people are clamouring for health care, so it is vital that the student nurse should also learn, at an early stage in her career, that it is not enough to be a good nurse. She must be a first class provider of nursing care. Except for a minor percentage, registered nurses will always be primarily concerned with the leadership of a team of less well qualified nursing personnel, for only in this way can our health needs be met. Their knowledge and skill must be put to work through others, and this implies professional skill and management ability of a high level.

Part of management effectiveness in the health services is knowledge and appreciation of the many professional subcultures found in the health services, the peculiar nature of role blurring, and the measure of cooperation and coordination that must exist between nursing and these groups. This is all part of basic management knowledge, and at an early stage the nurse must learn how to utilise such knowledge for the implementation of services. Her effectiveness will depend in some measure upon practical experience in this maze of subculture relationships.

Moreover, the expressive role of the nurse, whether in its broadest sense or limited to its narrow sense of rendering individual personal care to one patient, requires a substantial degree of management expertise if it is to be effective. Throughout it is the management concept which converts professional efficiency in nursing into professional effectiveness. A professional nurse is, in management language, a knowledge worker. She is the kingpin in the structure of health services, but she can be effective only so long as she is a true knowledge worker whose knowledge enables a herculean task to be done through the utilisation of the services of supplementary nursing groups and the incorporation of the principles of management at every level of activity.

In a limited learning situation, excluded from full departmental team work, the student is denied the rich and varied experience which responsibility for groups of patients provides. She does not learn to utilise the potential of co-workers above and below her in the situations which face full members of a departmental team, particularly in institutional practice. As a result she may find that institutional nursing, with its continuous demand for management ability, is beyond her and may move to less demanding fields of nursing or leave nursing altogether, because the educational system has denied her the opportunity to develop. It has taught her only the strength of the wolf and *not* the strength of the pack.

At the other end of the scale is the type of nursing education which believes that nursing can be learnt only by making the student nurse a drudge who is endlessly engaged in repetitive tasks without knowing the reason why. This school keeps theory to a minimum and applies rigid rules. The margin for human error is lessened by requiring slavish adherence to set rules. The stress is on 'how' and not 'why'. Needless to say, in such circumstances there is no room for the exercising of initiative and management is imposed from above without consultation with or garnering of ideas from subordinate ranks. This results in a restrictive, tradition-fettered situation and promotes the fallacy that all the brains are at the top, from whichever end one may be looking at the hierarchy. This has done immeasurable harm to the development of management potential in the nursing profession. It also helps to drive some of our best nurses from institutional nursing, for the intelligent nurse finds such a situation totally unacceptable. She declines to run with a pack which never gathers at the council rock and never draws out the full strength of the wolf (with apologies to Kipling).

Somewhere between these two concepts a balance must be struck. The commodity that nursing has to provide is effective patient care on a very broad spectrum to a very large number of people. It has to do this by defining its objectives, and by organising, directing and supervising human beings to achieve them. If the newly qualified nurse is unable to obtain the answers to the questions posed by Kipling's 'six honest serving men', *what, why, when, where, how, who*; if she is unable to coordinate the activities of a multidisciplinary group of workers and patients; if she is unable to meet contingencies for which no guidelines exist with the managerial confidence which such action requires; she will be a drag on the organisation which employs her.

It is imperative that even at the lowest level of nursing management the education of the future registered nurse must be geared to preparing her for the responsibility of running a department, be this institutional or non-institutional. The abilities and skills she will require cannot be learned 'in passing' at the bedside. Her responsibilities will embrace the establishment of objectives, the coordination of activities to achieve these objectives, the selection and direction of the persons to carry out the activities, and above all the capacity to get not only her own staff, but also personnel from other departments who contribute to the care of her patients, to work harmoniously together toward a common purpose. If she undergoes no basic management preparation as an integral part of her professional course, the achievement of really effective nursing care will be impossible.

With the expansion of health services the newly registered nurse will have very little time to learn the science and art of management from an immediate superior, such as occurs in the senior ward sister-sister situation. If the services are to be kept going, the newly registered nurse will inevitably take on the management of a department within months of qualifying. In this position she has to make a contribution to the total control of the organisation by expert management of the human and material resources under her jurisdiction. She also has to make a contribution to the pool of ideas from which top management draws.

A foundation in management education can readily be integrated into the basic nursing syllabus because modern nursing education provides (or should provide) a substantial core of study in sociology, psychology, social pathology, social economics in relation to health services, and social care. This forms a basis for an *elementary* course in the theory and practice of administration which deals with the meaning of the activity and the manpower, methods, materials, money and measurement involved. This could be taught in conjunction with an overview of the health needs of the community as a whole, the methods of analysing and meeting those needs, the methods for achieving high level management in each department and subdepartment of the organisation, and the role of each registered nurse in the total management situation.

Logical philosophies, attitudes and concepts and the ability to sift opinions, establish facts and put these down in a well-reasoned report that is clear, complete and concise are fundamental management attributes. So is the art of giving an order that is so specific that it cannot be misunderstood. The art of communication forms the very core of management. How to correct errors in others so that they are recognised without ill-will or resentment, how to spot personal errors of judgement, and how to remain abreast of developments in the work situation with confidence are all attributes which need to be founded and polished in the basic course.

Management training should be extended as a continuous process before the nurse is exposed to formal courses which lead to a qualification in management theory. This could be done by means of in-service education and through seminars, workshops and expert study groups. It would keep personnel on their toes and at the same time enable the controlling authorities to solve specific management problems and to learn what management problems personnel actually encounter.

Similary, basic management concepts should be taught as an integral part of all post-basic specialised clinical courses. An expert in a clinical speciality should be well-versed in management concepts so that she is able to balance the needs of patients in specialist services against the total needs of other, less specialised clinical services. This is consistently overlooked. A clinical nursing expert who lacks basic management knowledge is of limited value, for high level professional patient care is totally dependent on smooth organisation and the optimal use and control of human and physical resources.

In addition, if the health service authorities or some other public service authority organise periodic short courses which study particular aspects of management, and relate these to the problems in the health services, these will be highly beneficial, provided a multidisciplinary approach is maintained and the participants are also exposed to some community challenges from experts in services outside the health field to prevent too much in-breeding of thought. This is what nurses must fight for.

This type of development should serve to keep personnel open to new lines of thought and to new ways of coping with the day-to-day management problems encountered at first echelon and middle management levels. It should help to maintain that flexibility of mind which is so essential an attribute in candidates for top management training. This process will help to bring the cream to the top for selection for top management education, so that the high energy individuals, from whom sound leadership and management potential flows, can be kept on their toes and challenged just a little beyond their immediate capacity, thus strengthening their loyalty and sense of personal achievement.

At the same time such continuing education promotes that essential precept of good leadership, namely ensuring that there will be competent, dynamic leaders coming up the line. Success in this field is not automatic. It is the result of high quality action by enlightened, confident minds who take pride in producing successors and do not fear the upward thrust of competent future executives.

I have devoted a considerable amount of time to dealing with preparation for lower and middle management levels because I believe that this is the Achilles' heel in nursing management. No amount of instruction in the art of administration given only after completion of basic professional training as a nurse will totally relax the rigidity in concepts and attitudes produced by basic education systems which overlook the vital role that management principles should play in the provision of health care. Nor can it undo the effects of a system of professional practice in which the student in her formative years is subjected to inflexible rules in a system of practice where domination is the accepted truth and delegation is heresy. However much successful nurse administrators may differ regarding management education for nurses, and there is naturally divergence of opinion, all agree that this rigidity must go.

Traditional post-basic nursing schools unsuitable for higher management training

I have been asked whether formal courses in management training for qualified nurses should be given at diploma or at degree level. There is a need for both types. What is vital, however, is that such courses should be given to the young registered nurse as early as possible, and that they should be located in the type of school where the student can share some of the learning experiences with other professions. Advanced training should not be given in traditional nursing schools.

Experience has shown that where such education is given in the isolation of traditional nursing schools it results in propagation of inbred ideas and little more. What the management student needs is an infusion of new and provocative thinking so that she may develop the insight and skill to challenge the wisdom of a procedure or policy. New ideas, the audacity of new lines of thought and the impact of other approaches to management are all necessary if nursing management is to play its full role in the maintenance of health services. A multidisciplinary approach to the constructive consideration of health management problems is vital, or the nurse will merely be exposed to a readjustment of old methods and prejudices.

In the isolation of the majority of nursing schools it is not possible to bring together different categories of student personnel such as prospective hospital administrators, hospital accountants, medical administrators, hospital architects, public administrators, organisation and method experts, medical sociologists and others associated with the maintenance of the health services. Nor is it possible to expose the student fully to contemporary thought on the issues which influence social change and will influence her cooperation with other members of the total health team and thus the provision of health services at every level.

If top nursing management training is carried out solely within the confines of a nursing school, nursing management will not develop the full confidence that promotes the free exchange of views with other administrative heads without fear that the rights or status of the nurse administrator will be undermined. A multidisciplinary training ground can do much to enable different groups of management personnel in the health field to understand, respect and support each others' role. Where any redistribution of responsibility must be made it will tend to be approached in such a way that each segment of the service seeks to promote effectiveness in achieving the common end. Interdisciplinary communication in the health services will become effective only when top management personnel study the science and art of management in a multidisciplinary milieu such as a university.

Training for management should be at multidisciplinary centres

Depending on the availability of facilities, training in management which leads to a recognised administrative qualification should be given at health service interdisciplinary staff colleges, colleges of higher education, or universities.

There is room for all three types of qualification. There could be one to two year diploma courses and three year degree courses with provision for post-graduate education. Wherever possible, all candidates who are in possession of the necessary university entrance qualifications should follow a degree course, but progress should not be stultified because degree courses are not available. Diploma courses, which stress the value of seminars, discussion sessions and project work, and which provide tuition in the sciences basic to management theory, can and do play a vital role in management education for nurses provided a multidisciplinary approach is maintained.

Correspondence courses

The question of the value of correspondence courses in management training for nurses also arises. Such courses should be instituted to assist married nurses and personnel members in remote and isolated areas. It is imperative that the student is able to take a variety of subjects to serve as a background to the management course. In addition, she should be able to participate in summer or winter seminars/group discussions/ workshops so as to make contact in group discussions in a multidisciplinary context. This can be done for all the support subjects for a nursing degree and workshops on nursing management can even be organised.

Realism needed

Though full-time residential degree courses in nursing administration are desirable, the crisis in health manpower which appears to be world-wide makes it impractical to send personnel to university for full-time study of several years' duration. The output of management potential would be much too small. It is more practical to enable members of the personnel of each health service organisation to adjust their duty hours in such a way that they can undertake part-time study at nearby universities or colleges of higher education. Thus the student remains in the work situation, but is still able to study common core subjects with students from many walks of life, of many age groups, and from many disciplines. She will learn a great deal from life on campus about the social pressures which exist outside the health services, and about ways and means of reducing the impact of such pressures on the provision of health services.

Remaining in the job she will continue to grow with it, and will be able to put many of the concepts learned during her studies to the test of practical application on the job. This is important because, in the final analysis, intellectual leadership can flow only from a person who has learned how to place emphasis on the conceptual and the human skills of management rather than on the traditional technical skills, and who has learnt to translate knowledge into personal effectiveness in a real-life situation.

If suitable subjects are chosen this type of study for management will highlight the fact that while management incorporates many technical skills, it is above all a social process which emphasises the end and not the means, and which does this through recognition that this social process involves human personalities, relations, motives and attitudes with enduring emphasis on the maintenance of morale and on accountability to the community that must be served.

It is not imperative, although it is highly desirable, to introduce specifically designed diplomas or degrees for nurses – any degree or diploma with social or public administration as a major would be suitable. Today many education authorities are prepared to provide elective subjects in courses, provided that the common core content of the course substantially exceeds the elective subjects. Nursing administration could be introduced as an elective, and this would substantially reduce the cost of providing courses specifically for nurse administrators.

This approach is stressed because degrees in nursing administration are not widely available, and in any case they must include common core subjects. However, it is preferable that nursing degrees are instituted, for such courses have the advantages that the common core subjects can be chosen more carefully to give nursing administration the depth and breadth of a full major subject which extends to the doctoral level. This is why in Western countries the trend is to introduce nursing degrees.

In addition to post-basic baccalaureate degrees in nursing administration there is room for a master's degree in nursing administration and for degrees at doctoral level, for it is particularly at this level that true research ability is developed.

The concept now current among some nursing educationists that nursing administration as a functional subject should not be taught in post-basic degrees (that is degrees taken after the person has acquired a basic diploma in nursing at a hospital school), but that it should be reserved for study at the master's level, is debatable. First things must come first. The health services of the world need competent nursing management and it is our duty to provide training for this wherever we can, so long as we break out of the system of isolated education for nurses. Only a very small percentage of nurses will ever read for a master's degree, so we must keep our feet on the ground and look after the masses while making available to a select group the opportunity to go further. There are outstanding nurses with three-year hospital nursing school diplomas who have the ability to profit immeasurably from post-basic nursing degrees with a functional aspect such as nursing administration as a major. We overlook this source of potential management personnel at our peril. In a third world context effective management of health care services is the mainspring of health care provision. Insistence on a master's degree for nurse administrators will defeat the objective of providing effective nursing management.

Expatriate training not to be encouraged

It is highly desirable that each country should provide its own facilities for training nurses in management. Such courses should be tailored to meet the special social and administrative needs of the country concerned. The courses provided for the sophisticated services of economically developed countries will not be suitable for some of the economically handicapped countries. The nursing management courses in South Africa take due cognisance of this, although a tendency has been discerned which indicates that nurses who are able to obtain foreign funding wish to acquire such qualifications overseas.

Content of courses

Advanced courses in nursing management should enable students to study the applied elements of sociology, psychology, social economics, social administration, statistics, the methodology of demographic analysis and social surveys and general principles and methods of administration, and to relate all these to management in the nursing services. There are many health authorities who cannot see why nurses undergoing management training should study such subjects. They have this attitude because they themselves stand apart from the community and its influences.

Nursing management effectiveness and executive reality

The subjects mentioned will make very little impact on management effectiveness unless the student is able to analyse precisely what is meant by management effectiveness and executive reality in the nursing situation. This is the most difficult part of a course in nursing management, because nurses frequently embark on the course with a background of rigid traditionalism, or with over-sensitive attitudes to the prejudices or lack of understanding of nursing problems of some doctors, hospital administrators, health service trustees and politicians.

Such an analysis should involve the study of current philosphy about providing health services and should explore the ways in which the demand for institutional care could be reduced, for without such understanding full cooperation with other members of the health team will not be possible.

It should provide for understanding of the fact that hospitals and other health services are social artifacts which will inevitably be affected by what goes on in the society of which they form part, while at the same time they are instruments of social development.

Further, it should lead to the art of sifting facts relating to the organisation and the social milieu so that judgement, planning and action may be based on facts which are relevant and important.

Such an analysis should teach the student how to multiply her own abilities through others by helping them to draw on her knowledge or on that of her supervisors to expand their contribution to the service.

At the same time, it must highlight the fact that the pressures of work and of change will be such that she will have to acquire the art of giving prompt and accurate attention to the challenges she faces in her organisation and in the community if she is to avoid disorganisation of her service.

It will have to clarify such points as how to:

   (i) allot time
  (ii) analyse the strengths and weaknesses of personnel
 (iii) set priorities
  (iv) cut out irrelevancies
   (v) make optimal use of personnel and materials
  (vi) use meetings effectively
 (vii) communicate
(viii) foster teamwork
  (ix) develop herself and her personnel
   (x) make sound judgements against a background of dissenting opinions
  (xi) use conflicts constructively
 (xii) use research tools correctly and not succumb to the tendency to institute research programmes where there is merely unwillingness to make an unpleasant decision.

Such analysis should make the student aware of the steps she could take to make management right down the line an instrument for humanising hospitals and health services; fitting the organisation to the patients' needs and not the patients to the organisation. This requires urgent in-depth study by all would-be nurse administrators.

Above all, she has to learn that management does not mean power *over* people, but power *with* people. The following lesson should be learned early: management is something which is done for people, by people and with people, and, because of the diversity of human abilities and personalities, no cut and dried rules can be laid down. She must learn how to draw on the sciences basic to management theory, and by blending these with knowledge of the task at hand, develop the art of 'playing it by ear' and doing so effectively.

Teaching methods important

Bombarding a student with lectures is not the best way to give her a grounding in these attributes. Multidisciplinary seminars and the project method of teaching, together with a limited number of carefully selected lectures from experts, are more likely to lead to the type of development outlined above. Time to read, to think, to work out projects, to analyse existing practices, to identify contemporary pressure points and to record findings and conclusions in an unambiguous fashion, is essential. The art of contributing to nursing literature on management topics should be cultivated during such a course.

Conclusion

The acquisition of a qualification in nursing administration should serve as the starting point for a lifetime of study, particularly at the multi-disciplinary seminar level, with continual assessment of the impact of social change on the management of the particular situation with which the nurse administrator is concerned. Only in this way will the fetters of tradition be loosened, the need for change in nursing administration be identified, new ways of solving ever-changing problems be devised and the confidence necessary 'to embark on great and honourable courses with a sure hope and trust' be built up.

5

The future of the nurse administrator as determined by the relevance of her role and functions in the administration of the contemporary health care system

[A 1975 to 1988 perspective]

Introductory commentary

All health planners are agreed that hospitals and non-institutional health services are changing their organisational as well as their structural patterns. This is due to political policy and the ideology of free enterprise, as well as to advances in science, major politico-socio-economic changes and the expectations of the public and the health professions. The development of exceptional levels of professional expertise among all categories of health service personnel also contributes to such change.

The current emphasis on the cost element of providing health care and the rise of a very large cadre of hospital personnel involved in the management of health services who are not themselves health professionals, but seek the power and status of health professionals, are threatening the position of health professionals in the management arena. This applies not only to posts in the upper echelons of the service, but to every management post, including those at patient care unit level.

The nursing profession has given much attention to this development. Nurses believe that the quality and quantity of nursing care available to patients depends on nursing management expertise. Indeed, judgements about the quality of nursing care are based on nursing expertise, and upgrading the nursing service requires nursing expertise in the management of resources, both human and material.

What is needed is a corps of nursing management personnel capable of 'managing' the knowledge required for managing the service for patient care and for patient care itself. This group must take responsibility for converting new theories and ideas into applicable techniques and policies within the parameters of the politico-socio-economic climate, the policies of the health care authorities and the scarcity of human and material resources which arises for various reasons.

The thrust of this paper is that nursing management as a function of nursing is being threatened, and there is evidence that this is the case in many parts of the world. This has led to a strong belief among nurses that nurse administrators should strengthen their position through the acquisition of appropriate skills. Nurses are aware of the following:

(i) There is a need for general as well as specific education for the preparation of nurse administrators. Nurses require a knowledge and understanding of economics, basic accounting and budgeting, labour law and labour relations, business law, the principles of personnel management, psychology, statistics and the use and application of computers.

(ii) They must develop conceptual skills, including the perception and measurement of the work environment, the formulation and definition of problems, the application of knowledge, the development of expertise and understanding of the ways and means of acquiring and utilising resources. They must learn to develop alternative solutions and to make well-reasoned decisions. They must also learn to make 'decision reviews' – to analyse the facts which led to a particular decision and assess the results of the effecting of the decision.

(iii) Interpersonal skills (or human relations) constitute the most potent element of skill in management. Understanding human beings, their needs, aspirations and attributes, abilities and fears, is vital to good management. Managing human beings within a work situation is an art which makes unprecedented mental and physical demands on an individual. It entails working with people to achieve a set objective, and therefore interpersonal skills are very important. An assessment of one's 'value system' which tests one's beliefs, attitudes, concepts and assumptions is essential to successful interpersonal relations. It is necessary to learn to assess the culture and climate of the service one serves, to identify with the organisational objectives, to accept the role responsibilities assigned to one, to identify the areas of policy objectives which fall outside of one's scope and to develop the motivation to function as a well-adjusted member of the health management team.

A top level nurse manager needs to be recognised as an important member of the management team – the need for recognition is a human need which cannot be ignored.

Nursing administration (management) is in the hands of the profession itself. The quality of contemporary nurse administrators and the education provided for the next generation of nurse administrators will determine the future of this category of nurse. If she is not equal to the new and continually changing demands she will be replaced by a manager who is not a nurse, nor even a health professional! The future is in the hands of the present generation of nurse administrators.

THE ADDRESS

Introduction

The question whether a nurse should hold a top management position in a health care system has been raised frequently by health service administrators over the past two decades. The current belief among some administrative personnel and health planners in both South Africa and the USA is that the post of nurse administrator (or chief nursing officer) is not justified in the light of modern developments and changing approaches in the health care system.

This question has arisen because in many cases role changes to meet contemporary political, socio-economic and health care strategies have not kept pace with the changing demands and activities of the health care system. Clarification of the nature of the desired role changes is essential if obsolescence is to be avoided.

Kaladic (1962:1-5) pinpointed the question when she said:

the thought being expressed more and more lately is that the person who administers the hospital department of nursing need not be a nurse. Some hospitals, especially if they have had difficulty filling the position of director of nursing services, are beginning to develop a director of patient services who has had management preparation. An assistant manages the department of nursing from the aspect of professional nursing involvement. Such an arrangement emphasizes management skills, rather than nursing ability in line with the theory that the person who directs the department of nursing is essentially an administrator.

Kaladic (1962:1-5) confirms her support for this in her statement:

I firmly agree that the primary function of the director is that of hospital management, that the position is essentially in the executive management type of profession rather than in that of the nurse practitioner.

She does concede that it is 'of value to have had a nursing background', and states that the director (nurse administrator) of a nursing service 'represents one of the largest and most important jobs in the hospital field'.

Speaking at the same conference Smith (1962) warned against the tendency of nurse administrators to seek assistant hospital administrator status. She believes that the nurse administrator must retain her identity in the same way that the heads of pharmacy, dietary services and the medical services retain their professional status. She has a point. Many nurse administrators in South Africa would like to see the title 'chief matron' changed to 'deputy superintendent (nursing)'. Herein lies a threat to the continued use of nurses in such posts. The Board of the South African Nursing Association would prefer the term 'chief nursing officer', which emphasises that the control of a nursing service should be in the hands of a nurse because it is essentially nursing management, its primary objective being quality care for each individual patient/client (Smith 1962:11-16).

Nurse leaders debate this question frequently, for their analysis of health care delivery shows clearly that no health service can function effectively without management input from well-qualified, experienced nurses. At the same time they realise that the threat of obsolescence of such a post arises from the fact that many nurse administrators are not assessing their role and function correctly in the light of contemporary developments in the health care system. The result is that health planners, administrative officers and work study officers do not always obtain an accurate perspective of the role and functions of the nurse administrator and therefore advocate that these posts should be phased out.

The reasons given for phasing out posts of nurse administrator

Protagonists of the phasing-out approach base their arguments on such factors as the following:

(i) Many of the services previously managed or coordinated by the matron's department no longer fall under her control. Such services are now either self-contained and self-managing, or are performed to an ever greater extent by outside contractors, for example dietary services, uniform and linen services, maintenance of equipment and fittings and inventory services.

(ii) A centralised personnel department should control all staff records, undertake all activities for the appointment of personnel, and control the implementation of all personnel policies and conditions. The welfare section should cope with all personnel problems that cannot be handled at ward level, with direct referral to the superintendent where necessary. The personnel section should have a special staff development section for in-service and continuing education programmes for all categories of hospital/health personnel, and not only for nurses. The personnel section should have a special staff development officer in charge, and should be able to draw on personnel from all the disciplines to contribute to the development programme.

(iii) Clinical supervisors (presently known as zonal matrons) should deal with all nursing issues in their area where these concern patient care.

(iv) Where personnel policies or welfare aspects are concerned, the problem should be dealt with by the personnel department. If the problem concerns hospital policy, it should be dealt with at the level of the superintendent. All nursing personnel should be allocated *en bloc* by the personnel department to the various clinical supervisors for detailed allocation within their area. Student allocation should be done by the educational director, according to their educational needs and in consultation with the clinical supervisors.

(v) Control of all aspects of nursing education should be vested where it belongs, that is in the head of the educational programme.

(vi) Control of nurses' residences should be vested in house committees and in an officer who is directly responsible to the medical superintendent.

(vii) Consultant services could be made available to the medical superintendent, either by the allocation of a nursing consultant between a number of hospitals maintained by the same authority, or by means of a consultant who is made available by the nursing service division of the central controlling authority.

(viii) As a natural corollary to programme budgeting, the systems approach in organisation will take on more prominence. This will result in a considerable flattening of the hierarchical pyramid.

(ix) The increasing use of operational research methods and of electronic data processing equipment to supply management with the information it needs for decision making requires new management skills which need not be developed at every level of nurse management, but are important at the consulting level.

The views of leaders of the nursing profession in South Africa on the phasing-out theory

While nurse leaders agree in principle that the above statements are valid in that modern nursing management could, with an entrenched consulting status, devolve these responsibilities onto other departments, they cannot accept that the role of chief nurse administrator is redundant, no matter how satisfactorily all these other issues may be arranged. In services where this pattern exists they have seen a concomitant slowing down in decision making regarding nursing needs and required action and have witnessed the consequences of this.

They believe that the protagonists of the phasing-out process have entirely missed the point with regard to what the real function of the chief nurse administrator is, namely *to ensure that patients receive the quantity and quality of nursing care that they need, at the place and time they need it, and that this care should be free from safety risks. This is the core function of the nurse administrator. One has to be a nurse to identify all the above. Unless nurse administrators are prepared to see this core concept in its true perspective and unless they are prepared to shed all responsibilities that other personnel can do equally well or better, so that they may be able to devote more time to the increasing demands of their essential role, the post of nurse administrator or matron will become 'a bit of past history'.* The watchword is thus: change and prepare for more changes, or be phased out.

Quo vadis?

Before the question how the nurse administrator's role must adjust to contemporary and future developments and what this role should be in the period that lies ahead can be answered, it is necessary to examine the evolving structure of the health services. Change in the health care delivery system is currently a worldwide phenomenon. In the RSA the new Health Act No 63 of 1977 will have a profound influence on the structure of the health care delivery system. This Act emphasises the health of the public and provides for the wide range of activities necessary to achieve this objective. The comprehensive health service approach places the hospital at the centre of a health maintenance organisation consisting of a variety of institutional and non-institutional services, or a health 'conglomerate' as it is known in international circles. Apart from its traditional function of caring for the sick in a particular stage of the ill-health situation, its new functions include such aspects as serving as a resource centre for personnel in the non-institutional services, as an educational centre, as a data centre, as a monitoring centre, and as a research centre with regard to health issues, community needs and resources and the educational needs of health professionals. Its function as a sophisticated diagnostic and treatment and care centre for those conditions that cannot be handled effectively in the non-institutional health care system, and as a provider and coordinator of all health care in an area, will take on increasing importance in the years to come.

With the promulgation of the new Health Act a reappraisal of the role and functions of the nurse administrator is appropriate, for hers is a key role in the coordination of the projected comprehensive health service. The new Act does not provide for one, overall controlling health authority, but for a conglomerate system. Therefore the success of its provisions depends entirely on the insight, understanding, goodwill, cooperation and coordinating activities of the policy-making, medical, administrative and nursing personnel of the various authorities, at both the planning and the implementation levels.

If the premise that the main role of the nurse administrator, whatever the level at which she functions, is to manage the nursing service in such a way that quality nursing care is ensured within the constraints of the resources available and the particular local health needs and social situation, then such a post can be filled only by a suitably qualified and experienced registered nurse. Years of analysing the role and functions of the nurse administrator and the problems with which she has to deal entrenches the belief that the above premise is correct.

The conviction that it calls for a nurse with a great deal of clinical competence and knowledge, managerial and educational expertise, and knowledge of community health needs and resources is strengthened daily by the realities of the health care delivery system. These realities indicate that the incumbent of such a post should be a graduate nurse who has a great fund of nursing knowledge and who has been moulded and tested in the crucible of demanding experience. She must have acquired a large fund of modern management knowledge and an extensive network of modern management skills. A mere patina of management ability, as indicated by the silver bars on her shoulders, is not enough. New demands require new approaches, so that such a person should be appointed to the post by a merit rating system based on the new criteria and not as a result of the passage of time under a seniority dominated system.

The consensus among nurse leaders in South Africa is that the nurse administrator is (or should be) the following:

(i) *A leader*   Without the ability to lead effectively, the nurse administrator cannot serve in the modern health care system. She is the leader of the nursing team and must have the ability and drive to lead *with* people. She must have a disciplined mind which interprets findings in the context of contemporary technology and health and social patterns. The professional sophistication required for collaboration with other health professionals requires preparation at either post-basic or post-graduate nursing degree level. Knowledge of the administrative process, both in its generic sense and as applied in the organisation and management of nursing services, as well as knowledge of the nursing education process, sociology, psychology, public administration and the contribution of computer services, is of fundamental importance to the nurse administrator of today and tomorrow if she is to make the contribution to the development of the health services that the importance of nursing as an indispensable component of health care warrants, and indeed demands. Nurse administrators not only decide the future of their own role, but through their actions decide the future position of nursing in the health service structure.

(ii) *A member of the planning, implementing and evaluating team*   The ability to function as a team member on a peer group basis at this level is of great importance, for it is at this level that the innumerable activities involved in providing nursing care are slotted into the right place in the total effort by a multi-professional health team providing health care. The ability to develop and contribute to executive collaboration at top management level is of cardinal importance.

(iii) *An analyst of social indicators* The health care delivery system, and the nursing system which is an integral part of it, are at all times influenced by the social system in which they operate and by the social changes that take place and the community needs that become evident. The indicators that predict or confirm such changes are of the utmost importance to all planners in the health care system. Competence in analysing social trends and community health needs and in identifying social indicators that have relevance for the delivery of health care and hence for nursing are becoming increasingly important in nursing administration. Some of the problems encountered in nursing and in the health care delivery system as a whole are due to the lack of attention to this dimension of social organisation, or to a specific aspect of such organisation.

(iv) *A programmer of nursing care* She has to do this with due regard for the legal powers, responsibilities and limitations of the contributions of the various members of the particular health conglomerate, and in consultation with the policy makers, the medical, administrative and nursing personnel of the authorities who have to provide a comprehensive health service in a particular area or region. A master plan for the delivery of nursing services, whether in a hospital, a local authority service or in the non-institutional health services of the provincial services, or at a totally integrated level, requires vertical and horizontal consultation with a variety of health professionals. It requires communication channels and skills and the ability to coordinate. These skills are of crucial significance and require other knowledge and skills and activities identifying nursing needs, setting standards of care, drawing up job descriptions, identifying the knowledge and the skills required by personnel to provide this care, evaluating standards of care, determining priorities in the utilisation of scarce resources, identifying the restraints and capabilities in each programme of care, and planning to circumvent restraints and fully utilise available capabilities and strengths in any given situation are all core functions in any programming process. In this respect the increased use of clinical nursing specialists, in both institutional and non-institutional services, the use of generalists in both these services, and the use of subprofessional categories of personnel require expert clinical nursing knowledge, professional practice theory, recognition of interprofessional 'grey areas', and managerial skill to define and demarcate roles within a specific health care situation and within a rapidly evolving medical, technological and social situation.

(v) *A coordinator of nursing care* For economic reasons, and to bring about improvements in the quality of patient care, the trend is to assign clinical nursing specialists to a medical speciality with dual responsibility to the medical specialist team and to the head of the nursing service. Such specialists are responsible for expert planning, guidance, teaching and care contributions in the particular speciality to patients in the institution as a whole and to patients in the home-care situation attached to the hospital. Their services are not restricted to special wards. This requires a great deal of top level nursing knowledge and top level coordination of nursing care. This trend and the benefits flowing from it are jeopardised if the nurse administrator does not understand or is antagonistic, to this development. In addition, the Health Act provides for the development of health care programmes in which the hospital constitutes only one part. In such a programme the nursing service is one that is provided for the whole continuum of health care, for all age groups and all health aspects, and in a situation that is not bounded by the limits of the hospital grounds. Coordination of care at all these levels and for all phases of the health care continuum requires advanced nursing knowledge, experience, management skill, and a great deal of goodwill and belief in the ultimate objective – health for the people!

(vi) *A coordinator of health care*   The nursing service is the key element in the provision of health care at any level. It is the service that provides contact of the longest duration with the individual, family or group. Seeing that the services are provided by a health team, the majority of the services that reach the patient do so via the coordination of a nurse. Such coordination and team effort is not confined to action at the patient/client level. The heads of the various services have to plan together and coordinate their efforts to achieve effective health care. Even at the top administrative level such coordination is essential so that the groups concerned can know what support they can expect to receive from each other's services, how it will be provided, and what input they must pledge. Since all services impinge on the work of the nurse in some way, coordination and cooperation at the nurse administrator level is imperative. It is neglect of this fact that leads to interdisciplinary conflict.

(vii) *An expert evaluator of the quality of nursing personnel as a determinant of the quality of nursing care*   The quality of nursing personnel is a major determinant of the quality of nursing care. The personality of the individual nurse, and particularly of the nurse in charge of a unit, for example the ward sister, or the nurse in charge of a clinic or district service, is crucial in the provision of quality nursing care. Not only her personality, but her personal and professional philosophy, her attitudes, her preparation, and her knowledge and skills are decisive in how she fulfils her role. Although much of this is the product of the developmental years of the individual – the community she lived in, her family structure, her family's ethics and norms, the local mores and culture, the influence of community organisations and schools – the influence of peer groups and general professional development play a profound role. The influence of nursing schools, of other professions and occupations represented in the health team, of the leaders of the nursing profession and, in particular, of the nurse administrator in charge of the nursing service, play an important part in providing insight into acceptable professional patterns of behaviour. Quality nursing care is not possible if nurse administrators at all levels of a service do not give particular attention to the factors above, for administrative measures alone cannot provide quality care. Professional insight is as essential to this activity as the ability to understand human behaviour. Knowledge of the behavioural sciences without a deep understanding of professional practica and professional motivations, beliefs and constraints or of human motivation tends to reduce investigations in these fields to intellectual, mathematically orientated studies that end up in a pigeon-hole while the problem remains unsolved.

(viii) *An auditor and evaluator of the quality of nursing care and co-auditor of the quality of total health care* Quality assessment in a cost-conscious health and social system is today part of normal health administration practice. The quality assessment aspect of nursing management expands to interdisciplinary assessment of the quality of the total health programme.

(ix) *A designer of feedback systems* Definite feedback systems are essential to all operational activities. Without the information they provide about inputs, processes and outputs the service would stagnate, for feedback is essential for quality control, effective utilisation of all resources and assessments of community satisfaction. The nurse administrator must know how to devise such systems.

(x) *A problem solver* In all organisations problems arise due to a breakdown in some section of the system or to human failings, unexpected community needs, social and/or political change, cultural issues and economic tendencies. However the service needs persist and so a solution must be found, and after implementation of the solution feedback and evaluation are necessary. As the service grows in complexity the problem-solving ability of the nurse administrator must grow to keep up with it.

(xi) *A resolver of conflicts* As service situations grow and became more complex, new lifestyles emerge, new values and norms influence man's conduct and new patterns of collective bargaining and personnel problem-solving techniques emerge, employer/employee conflict situations will inevitably increase. At the same time interdisciplinary conflicts due to the growing number of grey areas between the various disciplines will accelerate, because professional groups feel threatened by other disciplines or some professions tend to extend their own range of activities and influence by deliberately encroaching on the terrain of other disciplines. Interprofessional conflict adds to the problem. All this affects the quantity and quality of patient care. Seeing that every aspect of care is either directly or indirectly affected by conflict in the health situation, the nurse administrator's role of conflict resolver in respect of inter-nursing conflict, nursing/other disciplines conflict and nursing/community conflict is reinforced by her role of coordinator to avoid areas of conflict.

(xii) *An analyst of nursing systems and a nursing systems designer* As the health care pattern changes to adapt to the changing needs of society, and as resources for providing health care become more scarce, a major activity of the nurse administrator will be to experiment with and to analyse new approaches to structuring the nursing system so as to provide the desired level of care within a socially and culturally acceptable and economically viable system. The preparation and implementation of appropriate nursing management, nursing care and nurse teaching systems are essential components of the development of a systems approach in the health service.

(xiii) *An analyst of data supplied by operational research programmes* For this activity the nurse administrator must have the ability to analyse data from mathematical and graphical presentations prepared by experts in data processing. Meaningful interpretation of such information is essential for decision making and for the preparation of reports.

(xiv) *A researcher* Without an ongoing programme of research into the various dimensions of the nursing service, effective decision making and progress are not possible. The nurse administrator needs to know how to plan and direct research into all aspects of the nursing process and how to identify issues that need to be investigated in a scientific manner.

(xv) *An analyst and purveyor of new knowledge* The nurse administrator cannot maintain her leadership role unless she remains abreast of developments in the health field, and in nursing in particular. It is not enough to keep up with technical knowledge only. She must keep abreast of trends in nursing and the health services at an international level so that she can maintain the vitality of the service she leads.

(xvi) *An expert at planning the financial needs of her department* Programme budgeting requires participation by all departmental heads in the budgeting process. The nursing service will stagnate if the nurse administrator is not able to identify needs and translate these into budgetary requirements, or is not able to present her case effectively.

(xvii) *An educator of health service personnel and of the recipients of health care* The management of formal nursing education courses is the function of the head of the educational institution offering the courses. The nurse administrator has a new and more dynamic role to play than she had in the past. Her role as a nurse educator should encompass such activities as the following:

  ☐ Identification of the formal educational needs of nursing personnel to enable them to fulfil their roles and functions. The person in charge of the service situation has a major responsibility to acquaint nurse educators with evolving practice requirements that will require amendments to the educational programme.

☐ Identifying the educational needs of practising personnel and meeting these needs in in-service and continuing education programmes. In addition, she has to assess how best to use human and material resources to provide such staff development programmes, and must establish, maintain and evaluate such programmes. Even if the in-service education section is under the control of the personnel division, she is still responsible for the following:

- collaborating with educational personnel in the evaluation of the clinical competence of basic and post-basic students and of pupil nurses, and in the establishment of criteria for such evaluation

- establishing and maintaining a climate conducive to learning for all health professionals associated with the particular service, and not only for nurses

- assisting with educational programmes for health professionals by ensuring that the facilities in the clinical situation are available to the students as and when required, that they receive an orientation to the role and functions of the nursing personnel, that they understand how the 'grey areas' between professions must be handled, that senior nursing personnel in the clinical situation contribute to the programme of the health professionals by precept and example and by one-on-one tuition for selected aspects (this is another coordinating function)

- ensuring that all nursing personnel know how to undertake patient/client teaching (health education) and what to teach in either the teachable moment or in organised patient/client teaching sessions

- identifying staff members' needs for advanced formal nursing education and taking steps to ensure that personnel are given the opportunity to obtain such education

☐ Acting as an advocate for the nursing personnel and for the patient. Her specialised knowledge obliges her to ascertain all the facts about a given nursing situation and to represent the needs of both patients and/or personnel to higher authority. In community circles she is also an advocate for nurse and patient.

WHO's views on the need for nurse administrators

WHO recommends that nurses should have:

the authority to plan and to administer the nursing component of the health services, and to participate as equal partners with heads of other professional and technical units in the formulation of policies, standards, objectives and plans for the development of overall health services and in the design of methods whereby these may be implemented and evaluated . . . a reliable, well organized system for collecting, analysing, interpreting, disseminating and utilizing data relating to nursing should gradually be established as part of the larger system of data collection for the health planning process (WHO 1972:5)

Nurses should be the primary users of this information in the health administration process.

In this paper the term 'nurse administrator' has been used instead of 'matron'. The two words which make up this term have a particular meaning. The letters of the word 'nurse' and the Latin origin of the word 'administrator' spell out the essence of the philosophy which should guide the nurse administrator.

N = Nearness to the patient/client and nurturing of his/her abilities to share in or take responsibility for the recovery and maintenance of his health

U = Understanding, unselfishness, usefulness and unity between the nurse, doctor, patient and other members of the health team

R = Realism, reason, reassurance, reserve about the patient's affairs, resourcefulness, research (what, why, when, where, how, who)

S = Service, self-sacrifice, self-discipline, self-assurance, support and sustaining of the patient/client and of fellow health workers, security for patients and staff

E = Expertise, example, empathy, education of patient and family, extension of the patient's ability to cope, education of personnel.

Administrator

In its literal sense the word derived from the Latin *ad-ministro*, which means 'I serve' or 'I minister unto'. Although in its modern sense it is interpreted as meaning 'managing', 'attending to', 'superintending', 'directing', 'controlling' or 'governing', the real meaning of the origin of the word should not be forgotten, but should nourish the attribute of humility.

This philosophy, which underlines the reason for the existence of nursing, spells out clearly that nursing administration is something within the purview of 'nursing' and not of general administration. It should clinch the argument as to whether there is a place for the nurse administrator or manager in the nursing service.

References

Kaladic, D. 1962. The director of hospital nursing service picks up the gauntlet. In *Blueprint for progress in hospital nursing*. Proceedings of 1962 regional conferences, National League for Nursing, New York.

Smith D. 1962. Nursing practice within a hospital nursing service. In *Blueprint for progress in hospital nursing*. Proceedings of 1962 regional conferences, National League for Nursing, New York.

WHO. 1972. *Report of the Inter-regional Seminar on the application of the planning process to nursing for nurse administrators at national level*. Geneva: WHO.

General references

Exodus chapter 18.
Notes on discussions with students on post-graduate courses.
Studies of the role and functions of nurse administrators in the RSA over a period of three decades.
Discussions at Congresses of the International Hospital Federation.
Discussions with professional colleagues in Europe, Britain, Canada and the USA.
The Health Act 63 of 1977.
WHO. 1968. *Hospital administration*. Technical Report Series No 395. Geneva: WHO.

Overview of the aspects dealt with in Part 2

The chapters in this section provide an overview of the thought on nursing administrators and their preparation for a period of three-and-a-half decades. Formal preparation of nurse administrators began in this country in 1951 with the provision of a one-year full-time (1½ years part-time) course leading to a diploma by a Hospital Services Department. Initially this diploma was not accepted by the SA Nursing Council for registration as an additional qualification, since it was the opinion of the leaders in the nursing profession that such a diploma should be followed only in Britain, where the Royal College of Nursing offered a course. The younger leaders of the profession objected to this, maintaining that the British course was tailored to meet the management needs of the National Health Service and was not suited to the nursing management needs of the health system in South Africa. Moreover, this restricted preparation to the select few who could afford to go to Britain.

After five years this qualification was recognised retrospectively by the SA Nursing Council. This is an example of the constraints which affected the emergence of a cadre of well-prepared nurse administrators. At that stage there was no educational institution prepared to provide this much-needed education for an important sector of the personnel of our health service. So, with the customary ingenuity of the nursing profession, financial assistance was secured, training venues were established, a curriculum was constructed, financing for students was obtained and a national examining body established (the SA Nursing Council). The next step was to move this training to universities and to phase out the Council's course, with the Council limiting its involvement to prescribing minimum requirements for recognition of the qualification for registration as an additional qualification. The phasing-out process has been a slow and costly one.

With the introduction of part-time post-registration nursing degree courses the development went a step further. Nursing administration was developed into a three-year major subject, with provision for advancement through Honours and Master's degrees up to Doctoral level. This development has highlighted the importance of the role of the nurse administrator in the health care system. It has also led to a desire on the part of academics in 'public administration' to absorb nursing administration into public administration. These academics tend to overlook the fact that a large number of nurse managers are now functioning outside the public service and occupy management posts in a wide variety of health services maintained by the private sector. *The key issue that is overlooked is that nursing management is about patient care, which requires clinical knowledge and competence, and which is permeated by nursing ethics and principles underlying the scope of practice of the nurse, as well as the acts and omissions of which the Council may take cognisance.*

The fundamental concepts of nursing administration have remained the same over three decades, but there has been a major shift in the depth of knowledge required and in the assertive, advocacy and executive aspects of the nurse administrator's role. The level of 'technical' knowledge required has also increased dramatically.

Because the majority of nurse administrators are women, the age-old issue of male-female ascendancy arises. This could be a factor in the subversive move to oust the nurse administrator from top management.

At the end of this century an assessment will have to be made of 50 years of nurse administrator preparation in this country, and of the evolution of the role. More research into various aspects of the role, functions and preparation will have been done. The research done thus far substantiates the views expressed in the chapters in this section.

The present generation of nurse administrators and how they adapt to changing needs will determine the ethics of nursing administration in the next century.

PART
3

Practice issues

6

The image of nursing – yesterday, today and tomorrow

[A current perspective]

Introductory commentary

Worldwide there appears to be concern about the image of nursing. A study of the literature indicates that research to validate the views held by the profession or the public about the image of the nursing profession is extremely limited and the findings are not applicable at an international level. It has been noted by the author that negative concepts of the image of the profession usually come to the fore when the profession is under continual stress. It is significant that in times of disaster or emergency an air of confidence, of absolute belief in its worth pervades the profession. Public praise at such times is always high. The profession sets itself very high standards and the leaders at all levels of the profession are always grieved and sometimes incensed, when one of its members gives way to human failings and has to be disciplined either by the courts, the SA Nursing Council, or both. At such times there is keen awareness that the image of the profession must suffer. The fact that the public disciplining of members actually enhances the profession's status in the community by reassuring the public of the profession's concern for its welfare is forgotten.

Nevertheless, there is cause for concern when poor quality nursing care puts patients at risk and members of the profession wear their uniforms in such a way that the dignity of the profession is called into question and trust in its efficiency and smartness is destroyed. Poor care of patients and their relatives and coarse behaviour in public result in a poor image of the profession. And often it is the little things that blot the image of a true professional.

When a nurse thinks and behaves like a professional, when she has earned the trust of her co-workers and the public, she has earned a positive image of nursing. Ultimately the image of the profession is in the hands of each individual nurse and her peers, who must ensure that she lives up to the standards of the profession.

The profession could enhance its image by letting the public know just how extensive and vital its services are. Why does it neglect to do so?

THE ADDRESS

Yesterday

The theme of my address is 'The image of nursing – yesterday, today and tomorrow'. I do not want to say too much about 'our yesterday', for this is well documented in the history of nursing. I merely want to remind you that in times of peace, war, disaster and epidemic, and in the everyday situation of coping with the health needs of the community, South African nursing has never been found wanting.

The nursing profession has produced leaders who have made an indelible impression on the life of the nation. In proportion to number they are the group of South African women who have received the most high honours, both nationally and internationally. They have made their mark as administrators, educators, clinical experts, researchers and writers. In times of crisis they were always in the vanguard of life-saving activities. I do not need to eulogise their doings. Look around you in Africa and recognise their contribution to the welfare of mankind.

Today

The nursing profession in South Africa has always had the courage to identify its shortcomings and to take steps to rectify that which erodes its development or undermines the quality of its care. It has always had the ability to identify its own weaknesses and the constraints within which it functions. Yet it has always lacked the drive to market itself, to let the nation know what its achievements are. It appears to be unable to 'sell itself' and to make the nation realise the magnitude of its contribution to the health care of the population. The news media pounce on the problem areas, but only very infrequently deal with some positive aspect of nursing or highlight the contribution to community welfare of that vast silent army of nurses who care for the nation's health, day in and day out, week after week, month after month, and year after year.

The extent of nursing's contribution

Few persons realise that during 1983 the small nursing force of some 60 000 registered nurses and some 80 000 subordinate categories of nurse had the unenviable task of providing health care to more than 31 000 000 persons (*Verslag* 1983:124-132). They did this under very difficult conditions, such as prolonged economic recession, with its massive unemployment; accelerated urban drift; civil disturbances; maldistribution of health care personnel; and lifestyle practices that are by no means conducive to the promotion of health. All these issues led to overcrowding in the health services at a time when, due to financial stringency, vacant nursing posts were frozen and nurses had to work extra hours without extra remuneration to cope with the workload. Despite the pressures in the work situation they managed to keep some 138 000 hospital beds and numerous clinics and day hospitals open, in the process providing several million days of in-patient nursing care, as well as coping with several million out-patient, clinic, day hospital and mobile clinic patient attendances, assisting with many thousands of operations, and delivering hundreds of thousands of babies.

The strain must have been wellnigh unbearable at times. Yet the main complaint of nurses during this time of stress was not their over-exhaustion, but their concern that their patients would not receive the quantity and quality of nursing care they needed. Although there were complaints about salaries, regulations and poor administrative practices, and although there was evidence of burnout, anger and disillusionment in the ranks of hospital nurses, the major complaints throughout this year, as they have always been, related to the nurses' concern about their inability to provide the quantity and quality of patient care they thought necessary.

The nursing profession in this country has much cause for self-congratulation for the excellence of the job it has done, and if the nation and its employers are not aware of this at least the profession knows what it has contributed to the well-being of the nation.

The profession needs to inform the public about its national contribution

Through its local branches the profession should inform the public about its aims, roles and annual contribution to the well-being of the nation. It should learn to publicise its role, what is stands for and how it aims to achieve its short and long-term objectives within a meaningful time span. If it is not prepared to do this it must accept the unenlightened views of the community about what nursing is and what its achievements are. This is an age in which the community perceives one's role and contribution in accordance with the way in which it is presented to the public. According to the concept 'perceptology', negative presentation leads to negative perception and negative interpretation of roles and achievements. The remedy lies in the hands of the profession.

How does the public perceive us? Grousing about salaries, hours of work, bad interpersonal relationships, uncaring doctors and a thankless public will not make the public aware of the importance of nursing in the life of the nation. Rather, proof of the indispensable multifaceted contribution of nurses to the public welfare will create this awareness. At the same time, it is the quality of care that John Citizen receives at the hands of the nurse, be she a Professor or Director of Nursing or a nursing assistant, that imprints a favourable or unfavourable image on the mind of the recipient of nursing care. The neatly groomed, competent, considerate, compassionate nurse who gives meticulous attention to basic nursing care as well as to high technology care, who through her general behaviour demonstrates that she is a cultured, well-spoken person, who respects the dignity and rights of the patients, his relatives and friends, and who cares for the beggar and the rich man, the terrorist and the policeman with equal skill and compassion, epitomises everything that is best in nursing. She epitomises true professionhood and demonstrates to the public that nursing is a caring profession followed by men and women of quality.

Peer group control is a cherished right

Despite the fact that the profession has made its contribution to the health care of the nation with quiet determination, dignity, devotion and a high level of professional competence, situations arise in which the public has to be protected against nurses. Human frailty being what it is, sometimes the profession, like any other occupation in the world, has to deal with those who fail to uphold its standards. Neglect of patients, acts and omissions which have ethical implications, and criminal action occur at times.

It is to the everlasting credit of the profession that such acts are not tolerated if they become known. Through its system of peer group control the profession institutes a public inquiry into alleged aberrant behaviour of nurses and midwives. It jealously guards this prerogative granted it by Parliament in terms of the Nursing Act. Through the peer group control system the profession guards against negligence and incorrect, criminal or other unethical practices. It exercises disciplinary control through punishment for negligence, incompetence or unethical behaviour. It concerns itself with protecting the public, on the one hand, and rehabilitating the transgressor, on the other. It exercises this difficult function with justice and concern for the well-being of the public and the good name of the profession, and with concern for its errant member. South African nurses can be proud of this system of legalised peer group control, which ensures orderly practice of the profession for the public good.

The profession has developed an excellent system of nursing education

The profession has reason to be proud of its system of nursing education. Despite innumerable problems, it has developed a system of nursing education that other Western countries are still struggling to achieve. Its university courses are well developed and of a high standard, and its nursing colleges are securely established in the post-secondary education system and are all associated with universities. Although its research programmes are in their infancy, a substantial amount of research has been done and is making a major contribution to the growth and development of the body of South African nursing knowledge. The profession has produced authors in a variety of nursing fields.

The profession has a place in the consultative process

Through its professional association the profession has attained a place in the consultative process for the planning and implementation of health services. It has done this at international, national, regional and local level, in both the public and the private sector. Many of its members have achieved high posts in the academic, administrative and clinical fields.

Nurses are involved in a wide range of leisure activities

Despite unfavourable working hours, in their leisure time many nurses participate in an extensive array of general cultural, historical, social, sporting, horticultural, artistic, environmental and community activities. They are involved in all aspects of human creative activity.

Nurses participate in the development of social services

Ever since the days of Henrietta Stockdale, the nursing profession has participated in, and frequently taken the lead in, the development of urgently needed health and social services. Overworked nurses of all ranks find time to give voluntary service to the Red Cross, Cancer associations, and care of the child, the aged and the physically and socially handicapped. Many are involved in health promotion and emergency care and support in their own neighbourhoods.

Tomorrow

The need to be alert to changes in society

We know our worth, but that is not enough. We have to be alert to the issues that arise as a result of changes in society and out of the provision of health care and manpower production. As this century draws to a close numerous issues will necessitate changes in the way that the profession adapts to evolving social circumstances, and in the way it handles its affairs. Analysis of judgement of the impact of current social forces and adaptability to change will play an important part in the survival of nursing as a force in the health care systems of this country.

Current issues urgently requiring study

There are numerous current issues demanding immediate scrutiny and action. These are primarily issues which affect the profession itself. Nevertheless they are vitally important, for if left unanalysed and undirected into positive action the profession will undoubtedly be substantially weakened. Some of these issues are common to nursing throughout the world.

There is time for only a brief look at a few of the more clamant issues.

Changing perspectives in health care

Constitutional change in this country, as well as the policy of massive privatisation of health services, will have a profound effect on the provision of health care and on the main providers of health care – the nursing profession. It will take a considerable time for health planners and health professionals to sort out the innumerable problems that must inevitably arise in the implementation of the new system of decentralisation of health services and the philosophy of integrated health services.

Insecurity of personnel, resistance to the implementation of new systems, and uncertainty about service demarcation are inevitable problems which will require considerable skill and goodwill to sort out. The nurses in leadership positions will have to be people who are trusted by the rank and file of the profession to ensure that nurses are enabled to provide an optimal level of nursing service while being assured of their own situation in the still unclear health policy situation. Privatisation of health care poses innumerable problems for the profession. These problems must be examined before large-scale privatisation becomes operative. Such matters as compulsory pension funds, revision of vacation and sick leave provisions, the institution of suitable career ladders, nurse administration *vis-à-vis* lay administration, doctor and nurse relationships in the private sector, the usurping of nursing functions by non-nursing personnel, the maintenance of standards of care when the profit element becomes the dominant issue in the care situation, surveillance of standards of care in the private health services and the contribution of the private sector to health manpower production are all issues requiring immediate attention.

Careful analysis of the facts and skillful models of the implementation of the desired practices must be made before there is large-scale introduction of private health services. Nurses must understand that the health plan makes provision for health care for all citizens – those who can afford to pay, those whose payment for services is via medical aid schemes and those who are semi-indigent or indigent and who are provided for by the state. The role of the profession is to act as watchdog to ensure that everybody in need of health care receives such care, and to bring it to the notice of the Department of Health and Population Development where serious shortcomings exist. Constructive advice and a willingness to cooperate in meeting the deficit in health care are the primary requirements in this regard.

The human rights theory that every human being has a right to health forces the nursing profession to assist in the education of the individual, the family and the community at large to protect and promote their health through safer lifestyles and responsible collaboration with health professionals. The profession has a key role to play in educating the public about family planning, nutrition and promotive and preventive health services so that personal decisions can be made on the basis of knowledge and trust. Above all, it must play the primary role in ensuring that the authorities provide facilities for the early detection and treatment of ill-health, and that such services are accessible to the consumers of health care. This it must do by means of negotiation.

The profession has a duty to involve itself in community planning, development and public policy formulation through service on commissions, councils, committees and in Parliament.

The increase in the multiplicity and multidimensionality of the problems in the health care system requires understanding by the profession and cooperation at numerous levels so that the aim of every professional nurse for personalised patient care can be realised.

Increase in interprofessional relationships

The increase in the multiplicity of interprofessional relationships in the health care system is resulting in the overlapping of the functions of the various disciplines represented on the health team. To avoid discord and prevent status-seeking conflicts among the members of the health team, the profession should ensure that its demarcation of the nurse's role is open-ended. It should also ensure that the profession is equipped to meet other health professionals at a level of competence that will ensure collegial cooperation. This is of crucial importance to the effective use of nurses.

Recognition of the nurse's role as social developer

The profession has to ensure that the role of the nurse as a social developer is recognised. Health care forms an integral aspect of the social development of an area.

The profession has a major role to play in identifying health needs, advising on the distribution and adequacy of coverage of available health facilities, evaluating the effectiveness of health intervention measures, the observable benefits derived from the utilisation of resources, the acceptability of the service to the community, the extent and potential of community involvement and the availability of local resources, and determining the reasons for escalations in costs, the nature of public expectations, the changing epidemiological pattern, the economic developments in an area and the questions that must be answered.

The image of the nurse

The profession must realise that the nurse practitioner's image is very important. She must be knowledgeable, competent, considerate and compassionate and her integrity must be beyond question. She must be a well-educated person who commands the respect of and can hold her own with other health professionals and the community. She must be a leader in every situation in which she works.

The need to understand and accept change

The profession must be constantly on the alert to adapt to change. This requires problem-solving ability, but also the credibility to initiate change. The profession must have honesty of purpose and self-confidence and be *au fait* with the situation to be changed and devoted to the interests of those who will be affected by change – the nurse and the patient. The profession must realise that change in the social and health care systems is an ongoing activity. Societal change and the dynamics of the interface between the various health professions and of the interface between the nursing profession and the consumers of health care and the health care authorities lead to change which might be destructive, but if correctly handled could be of inestimable value to all concerned, particularly the receivers of health care. Constructive change in the health care situation derives from constructive assertiveness by the health care professions on behalf of those whom they serve. Effective identification and analysis of problems, constructive decision making and effective communication are the tools the profession has to use to carry out its task.

The use of professional power

Professional power must never be used to the detriment of the patient. Negative wielding of professional power is misuse of power. Wisdom and the awareness that the nurse has to serve all mankind, irrespective of his political or religious persuasion, requires the profession to deal with problems solely on the merits of the case and not to be influenced by political considerations. Persuasion through the use of reason rather than threats is the most powerful and most civilised way of wielding power. Change in a democratic organisation relies on well-reasoned persuasion. All health professions are really 'persuasion professions'. Simons (1976:133) believed that all professional practitioners 'have an ethical obligation to acknowledge their roles as persuaders'. Silvey (in Lancaster & Lancaster 1982:134) states a fundamental truth:

> I would define persuasion to be the single encompassing term in any process of communication which influences thought, belief, attitudes and for behaviour.

Growth in the number of subprofessional personnel

One of the most urgent problems faced by the profession of nursing is the increase in the number of subprofessional categories of nursing personnel. At present there is a ratio of registered nurses to enrolled and assistant nurses of 1:1,5. This is a serious matter. The quality of care that the profession can provide depends on the availability of registered nurses. The imbalance of personnel has become an issue worldwide. The International Council of Nurses (ICN) has taken a stand on this.

The ICN considers the existence of three categories of nurse to be undesirable. Great Britain is revising its approach at present. It proposes that nursing shall be done by registered nurses, assisted by hospital auxiliaries (who are not nurses) to do non-nursing duties. To this end it is updating the training of enrolled nurses so that they may become registered nurses. Those who are not able to benefit from such a course will remain enrolled nurses until their retirement. This is an issue that the profession in South Africa needs to examine, for there is evidence that the imbalance between registered nurses and the enrolled categories is growing rapidly.

Know your standpoint

To be an effective persuader one has to have a total belief in one's standpoint. One cannot sell an idea which one does not wholeheartedly support. Belief in one's standpoint gives it credibility.

Why are we so ineffective in selling nursing's vital role, in making the community aware of our achievements? Is it because we do not have enough trust and belief in our profession?

Let us explore this thorny statement!

References

Lancaster, J & Lancaster, W (Eds.). 1982. *The nurse as change agent*. St Louis: Mosby.
Simons, HW. 1976. *Persuasion: Understanding, practice and analysis*. Menlo Park, Ca: Addison Wesley.
Verslag van die Wetenskaplike Komitee van die Presidentsraad oor Demografiese Tendense in Suid Afrika, 1983. PR/1983. Staatsdrukker: Pretoria.

7

Nursing practice – reality or dream?

[A current perspective]

Introductory commentary

There is a great deal of misunderstanding of the concepts 'nursing practice' and 'nurse practitioner'. This arises from the use of these words in American nursing culture, where the legal status of the nurse and ideas about what constitutes a practitioner are considered against a background different from that prevailing in South Africa. This is an issue which can be assessed only within the context and practices of a particular country.

South African nurses do infinite harm to the cause of nursing in South Africa by lifting concepts from American literature without analysing the meaning of such concepts in the South African context. The American literature is extremely valuable for indicating to the nurse the diversity of legal connotations of nursing in the world and how careful one has to be in giving a designation to a particular professional activity.

It is frequently found that nurses in third world countries have been prepared as 'nurse practitioners'. Sometimes an adjective precedes this term, for example, 'family nurse practitioner' and 'primary health care practitioner'. This creates the impression that other registered nurses and registered midwives are not practitioners, that they have not attained the exalted status of 'nurse practitioner'. The fact that in South Africa midwives have been legally recognised practitioners since 1652, and nurses since 1891, is overlooked. It was 'independent nurse practitioners' who campaigned for state registration for nurses in the former Cape Colony (now the Cape Province of the Republic of South Africa). The adjective before the words 'nurse practitioner' merely designates a particular category of nurse practitioner.

This issue has a major effect on how the ethos of nursing is viewed by both the profession and the public. A proper understanding of the ethos of the profession has its foundation in a clear understanding of the concepts 'nursing practice' and 'nurse practitioner'.

THE ADDRESS

Introduction

For the purpose of this presentation, the term 'nursing practice' excludes 'midwifery practice'. The debate as to whether a nurse is a practitioner or not centres on the nurse, and not on the midwife. Both legally and by customary practice, in South Africa midwives have enjoyed the status of practitioner since 1652, while nurses have been recognised as legal practitioners only since 1891.

Nursing practice a reality

The thesis of this presentation is that nursing practice is a legal and a social reality, and definitely not a 'dream'. It is a phenomenon that exists as an extrenched part of the social structure of this country and is recognised in law. What we make of practice determines the reality of it from the point of view of the community.

The concept 'practice'

Exactly what is meant by the term 'practice' when it is used in a professional context? *Webster's* dictionary describes practice as follows: 'to put knowledge into practice, to work at, or to follow a profession'. The *Reader's Digest Illustrated Dictionary* refers to practice when used in a professional context as 'the exercise of an occupation or profession'. Neither of these authoritative sources defines how the occupation or profession is to be practised. In other words, the concepts inherent in these definitions apply equally to 'private practice' and to 'practice in an employment situation'. For most professions private practice was essentially a phenomenon of the 18th and 19th centuries. Today, worldwide, more professionals practice within an employment situation than out of one.

Some misunderstanding is evident

There appears to be a measure of misunderstanding about what is meant by 'nursing practice'. Some American nursing literature views practice in the same way it is viewed in South Africa (ANA 1973:Preface). However, some authors appear to adopt the standpoint that one practices nursing when one is engaged in 'private practice', that is when one conducts an independent nursing 'business'. A nurse practitioner treats patients and advises clients referred to her by a medical practitioner, or who come without referral to obtain a specific type of nursing care. (Jacox and Norris 1977:xiii, 3:21, 22, 23, 25, 193, 198, 207). There is frequent reference to the emergence of a new category of nurse known as a 'nurse practitioner'.

The need to be specific

There is a need to be clear in one's writings and discussions about the meaning of 'nursing practice' within the national context. It is desirable that the SA Nursing Council should publish a national statement in which it makes it clear that the only valid definition of nursing practice for South African purposes is that provided in the Nursing Act. However, it appears that nurses do not study the Nursing Act in order to clarify their practitioner status.

Three points of view on the topic of this address

The question 'nursing practice – dream or reality?' can be approached in three ways, namely in terms of the legality of nursing practice, in terms of the fulfilment of a practitioner role, irrespective of the health care setting in which the nurse functions, and from a care point of view.

The legality of nursing practice

In South Africa nursing practice is a legally entrenched concept which has the same validity, and hence the same reality, as the practice of the medical practitioner.

The legal practitioner status of nurses in South Africa dates back to 1891, when the provisions of the Medical and Pharmacy Act No 34 of 1891 provided for the registration of medical practitioners, dentists, apothecaries (including chemists and druggists), midwives and nurses on the same register, although in different sections thereof. Section 47 of this Act specifically provided that registered persons who were found guilty of infamous or disgraceful conduct in any professional or other respect, after due inquiry by the Council, were to have their names removed from the register, subject to approval by the governor, and once this had been done they were not entitled 'to practise their profession'.

Inherent in every section of this first Act, which provided for the registration of these five categories of health practitioner, was the principle that the person observes the law and its regulations to retain the right to practise his/her profession.

The Medical and Pharmacy Act of 1891 showed clearly that registered health professionals were dependent on observance of the law to remain in practice. Nowhere was there any mention of nurses being dependent on the orders of doctors to practice their profession. Personal responsibility and accountability, which lies at the core of professional practice, was inherent in every aspect of the Act and its regulations.

Section 31 of this Act specifically provided for the withdrawal or cancellation of a certificate of registration granted to a trained nurse if it was proved that the holder was grossly incompetent or had been guilty of such improper conduct as in the opinion of the Council rendered it inadvisable that she should 'continue to practise as a trained nurse'.

Nowhere in the regulations gazetted under this Act did it appear that nurses could practise their profession only in an employment situation, or under the supervision of doctors. The regulations treated nurses as independent practitioners on the same lines as the other four categories of persons registered in 1891 were treated.

It could not be otherwise. There were very few hospitals at that time and the major part of health care was provided by nurses in the homes of their patients. These were 'self-employed' nurses or nurses in 'private practice'. Wherever medical assistance was available they worked in close collaboration with the family medical practitioner in the same way that they worked closely with the doctor in the hospital situation. Mutual interdependence was well-entrenched. Up to the beginning of the South African War, 1899-1902, the majority of registered nurses were in private practice. Some had 'rooms' in their homes from which they provided a service, others undertook private nursing, and some established small private nursing homes. These nurses established a network of small hospitals and home care facilities which became the foundation of the health services which exist today. The practice of these private nursing practitioners helped to broaden the scope and range of medical practice.

At the same time, institutional nursing practice was becoming entrenched. A study of the letters, documents, diaries and books written by medical practitioners indicates that by the end of the 19th century the trained nurse was established in Southern Africa as a registered practitioner with a whole range of independent functions. These were:

(i) supervising the patient and his immediate environment

(ii) observing the signs, symptoms and reactions experienced by the patient

(iii) recording the symptoms, signs, reactions and treatment and care given

(iv) supervising and directing the subordinate personnel serving the patient's needs

(v) coordinating the services of other workers who serve the patient's needs

(vi) planning and implementing independent patient care activities such as nursing care and supportive care, the maintenance of personal and environmental hygiene directly associated with patient care, health education and assistance with social services

(vii) personal responsibility and accountability for all her own acts and omissions, including the carrying out of any prescription or request from the patient's doctor provided this was within her range of competence and was legal, clear, accurate and not against the policy of the authority who had a contractual relationship with the patient for the safety of his person, his name and the property he brought with him on admission to the hospital. She had the right to refuse to cooperate with the doctor if such cooperation was against her religious beliefs and had a clear duty to protect the patient against illegal and incompetent health care, and from the medico-legal hazards found in hospitals.

Legislation enacted in Natal in 1899 was similar to that enacted in the Cape. It is interesting to note that when Natal first commenced training nurses in 1890, the regulations of the hospital provided that probationer nurses had to give an undertaking that they would follow the orders of the doctors meticulously and be subject to him at all times. This provision was not entrenched in the first law and regulations which authorised state registration of nurses and midwives in Natal. Nevertheless, we may presume that this concept was carried forward into the 20th century.

After the South African War (1899-1902) the Transvaal and Orange River Colonies enacted legislation similar to the Medical and Pharmacy Act of 1891. It is interesting to note that the word 'medical' was considered a 'generic' word which included medical practitioners, dentists, nurses and midwives.

It is clear, therefore, that by the beginning of the 20th century registered nurses in the colonies now constituting the Republic of South Africa were practitioners in their own right, no matter where they worked – in private practice, in hospitals, in the military services, or in doctors' consulting rooms. On the grounds of this professional practitioner status qualified nurses were given 'officer status' during the South African War.

If this was the status of nurses at the turn of the century, what went wrong? This question is asked because for many years during the 20th century nurses subjected themselves to a situation in which they negated their legal rights as practitioners. Yet legally they were involved in a cooperative practice situation, with both doctor and nurse jointly and separately responsible for 'their patient'. Nurses practised their profession within the ambit of statutory laws and regulations, the common law, and the unwritten code of their profession, yet they abrogated their status as practitioners.

A factor of major importance in the changing attitudes of nurses, attitudes which made them subservient to doctors (even if the law did not place them in such a position), was the advent of the South African War. Large numbers of nurses from the Poor Law hospitals in Britain served in the war. Many remained in this country to help with the reconstruction of the health services. They became matrons and sisters in the hospitals and the British pattern of nursing became established practice. At that time Britain had not yet acquired legislation to regulate nursing practice. A new concept of doctor-nurse relationships became entrenched in South Africa and the concept of the nurse as a practitioner in her own right disappeared for a time. It was held that the nurse was in the hospital to carry out the doctor's orders.

At the same time successive economic recessions caused nurses to seek employment in hospitals, where the bureaucratic machine and fear of job losses during a time of great financial hardship smothered ideas of independent professional practice.

Nursing education developed as a by-product of hospitalisation. It was geared to the requirements of the bureaucratic system and the orders of the doctor. Lectures in the theory of nursing amounted to a study of the basic sciences and of diseases. Lectures were given by doctors and the matrons and sisters gave demonstrations of the procedures used in nursing. There was no true preparation of a professional practitioner. Qualified nurse tutors were introduced in the early twenties, but they had received their education overseas in a milieu in which the philosophy of doctor supremacy in the nurse-doctor relationship was rampant. As a result of this the education of several generations of South African nurses reflected the concept that the nurse had a function dependent on the doctor, and that the nurse (as opposed to the midwife) was not a practitioner. Yet, as late as 1944, the certificate issue by the South African Medical Council to a registered nurse clearly stated that she was competent 'to practise' as a medical and surgical nurse.

The concept of the nurse as a practitioner and the principle of professional practice are securely entrenched in the Nursing Act No 50 of 1978, and in the Nursing Acts preceding this. Despite these legal provisions it has been a dispiriting task to make some nurses realise that they are legal practitioners, fully accountable for their own acts and omissions and jointly responsible with the doctor for patient care.

Fulfilling the role of practitioner irrespective of the health care setting

The law empowers the nurse to practise her profession in any type of health care situation. The parameters of such professional practice are competence, authority, responsibility, accountability, independent decision making, collaboration, facilitation, advocacy, nursing diagnosis, planning of nursing care and recording of actions on behalf of the patient/client.

One of the constraints on nursing practice in the hospital situation is the fact that we call the division responsible for nursing care the 'nursing service department'. Emphasis falls heavily on the concept 'service' in a bureaucratic sense. It is an integral aspect of a bureaucratic hierarchical organisation. This constitutes a threat to professional responsibility and professional practice concepts. Take a close look at the 'nursing service' concept as evinced in many of our hospitals.

It is not service to the patient, but 'service to the service organisation' that lies at the centre of nursing practice in many of our large institutions. It is the duty of every nurse manager to ensure that the registered nurses on her personnel are true practitioners. They must be freed from the excessive bureaucratic restraints that make them service automatons, and they must be helped to act as fully accountable practitioners. It is ironic that the only time that the health care authorities stress the professional accountability of a nurse is when a claim for damages is lodged by a patient. Is it not time to call existing nursing service divisions 'nursing care divisions' so as to ensure that the emphasis falls on the professional practice aspects of the nurse's contribution to patient care and the centrality of the care of the patient is emphasised?

The concepts 'nursing practice' and 'nurse practitioner' were undermined by matrons in the organisational hierarchy. Now only nurse managers can lift nursing practice to its rightful status in health care institutions. The quality of nurse managers and their insight into the management of professionals can resolve this contentious problem.

This is a vitally important problem. Nurse leaders have a duty to ensure that their professional nursing personnel practice as professionals. That is the whole justification for the nurse manager being a professional nurse, for presumably she knows what the professional practice of a nurse entails. If she continues to negate this vitally important dimension of her work the end result will be that a nurse manager need not be a professional nurse, for nurses will not be concerned with professional practice, but only with carrying out the rules of the institution and the orders of the doctor.

The choice is ours. Will we make professional practice a reality, or will we live in a dream world and continue to pay lip service to the concepts professional practice and practitioner status?

The reality of nursing practice

While the legality of nursing practice is very much a reality, can we say the same about nursing practice itself? How nursing practice is carried out constitutes an experience for the patient and his family. Is the reality of nursing practice what the patient expected?

We all know that some neglect of patients occurs daily and that slovenly, indifferent and even ignorant practice occurs at times. We see untidy nurses in the wards and on the streets. Are we looking facts in the face and admitting that our nursing practice is not all it should be in all centres? Is the profession aware of the number of nurses who face disciplinary action by the SA Nursing Council annually? Are all of us prepared to 'walk the extra mile' when the need is great? How many of us share in the work of our professional association? Are we really professional practitioners if we disregard this vital element of our professional life? Do we all behave like competent, knowledgeable professional practitioners in our collegial relationships with other members of the health team, or do we take a back seat when professional case discussions are held? Do we shrink from the professional limelight and behave as if we are ashamed of our existence as professional nurses?

If a nurse does not understand the basic legal, ethical, physical, biological, therapeutic, social and psychological elements of safe and considerate nursing care, if she does not understand her own rights as a registered nurse practitioner *vis-à-vis* her employer, if she does not understand or comply with the fundamental principles underlying the professional conduct of a registered nurse, if she does not understand and observe the nature of her responsibilities as a colleague of the doctor, if she does not understand or accept that the patient is her patient as well as being the patient of the doctor, if she does not understand or accept the rights of the patient in the care situation, and if she has no confidence in herself as a practitioner, we cannot call her a professional practitioner, no matter what the law says.

Professional practice is based on knowledge, understanding and acceptance of a role, responsibility and accountability, and if the nurse does not know or observe the principles enumerated in the preceding paragraph, there is no professional practice. Under such circumstances practice is an illusion and reality is shrouded in ignorance, with negation of professional responsibility. We may say that this type of practice is a dream of the kind known as a nightmare! Both the community and the profession are at risk.

Conclusion

We know the problems we are facing. The real question is what are we going to do to make nursing practice safe and satisfying for all those who seek our help? What are we going to do to make every nurse practitioner a practitioner in the fullest sense, so that nursing practice may bring real meaning to the life of the practitioner?

If we believe in nursing practice we have a duty to help our fellow practitioners to be competent and compassionate practitioners. The ball is in our court!

References

American Nurses' Association. 1973. *Standards of Nursing Practice*. Kansas City: ANA.

Jacox, AK & Norris, CM. 1977. *Organizing for Independent Nursing Practice*. New York: Appleton-Century-Crofts.

Medical and Pharmacy Act No 34 of 1891. Colony of the Cape of Good Hope.
Medical, Dental & Pharmacy Act No 13 of 1928. Union of South Africa.
Medical and Pharmacy Act No 21 of 1899. Colony of Natal.
Medical & Pharmacy Ordinance No 1 of 1904. Orange River Colony.
Medical & Pharmacy Ordinance No 29 of 1904. Transvaal Colony.
Mundinger, M. 1980. *Autonomy in Nursing*. Germantown: Aspen Systems Cor-
    poration.
The Nursing Act No 50 of 1978.
The Nursing Act No 45 of 1944.

8

Communication: the basis for quality
nursing practice

[A 1983 perspective]

Introductory commentary

It is a sad commentary on the education of nurses and midwives that while they are technically very competent, there is considerable room for improvement of their communication skills. This is reflected in the numerous problems they encounter in verbal communication with their patients and their relatives, the general public, their employers, their subordinates and other members of the health profession.

Poor communication in writing leads to problems regarding the maintenance of patient records, the writing of reports and correspondence with professional associations and the South African Nursing Council. Furthermore, professional practice loses out in that too few nurses prepare papers for publication or for presentation at professional or interprofessional seminars and congresses.

The nursing profession is giving considerable attention to the problem of poor communication in nursing. How it is approached will have a major impact on the ethos of the profession now and on what it will become by the turn of the century.

THE ADDRESS

> Word is not crystal, transparent and unchanged;
> it is the skin of a living thought and may
> vary greatly in color and content
> according to the circumstances and the time
> in which it is used.
>
> Oliver Wendell Holmes

Introduction

I want to deal with the question of communication as the basis for quality care from three points of view – those of the system, the top nurse manager and the person-in-charge of the ward, department or clinic. In restricting my discourse to these three levels I am by no means implying that effective communication in the health care system is not the concern of every worker and also the patient/client.

Of necessity each aspect can be dealt with only very briefly, although it is possible to produce a number of textbooks on each one. Because the quality of nursing care is part of the quality of the whole system of health care, I specifically want to highlight the following aspects:

(i) communication as the bond of humanness in the health care system

(ii) communication as the essential element of nursing administration
(iii) communication as the essence of interpersonal relationships.

Communication the basis of all relationships between all living things

The basis of all human relationships is communication. Indeed, communication is the basis of all relationships between all living things. Only man is capable of the rich diversity of sounds, symbols, actions, attitudes and thought projections which have enabled him to obtain mastery of the known world and have opened the gateways of the universe for exploration. Everything that man is able to achieve arises from the priceless God-given gift of communication. To be able to communicate is the very essence of living. The very meaning of the word illustrates the importance of the concepts inherent in it. The word derives from the Latin *communicare*, which means 'to share', 'to impart', 'to take part in', 'to join', 'to connect', 'to unite'. *Communication is the bond of 'humanness' that makes man one with his fellow men.* It is the cement which stabilises his existence within his family, social group, community, nation and the world at large. It is the means whereby man makes his place in the world and proclaims what he is and what he wishes to be. It can be the most positive and also the most negative experience to which a human being is subjected.

Man communicates in many ways – through speech, the written word, posture, actions, achievements, failures, looks, grooming and dress, expressions, lifestyle, work, possessions, the place he lives in and many other overt and covert activities based on his rich cultural heritage. Communication is not only man's way of expressing his humanness and dignity, needs, strengths and objectives and concern for his fellow men, but constitutes the very bricks and mortar that build civilisations.

Indirect communications from the system affect the quality of nursing

What are the unwritten and unspoken forms of communication which flow from the 'system' and have a profound influence on the quality of nursing and of all aspects of health care? I want to focus your attention on only a few issues which show more clearly than words the measure of concern that emanates from a particular health system. Concern is the basis of quality care.

Every aspect of the *policy* of a health care system is a form of communication, not only to those who have to implement the policy, but also to those who receive the health care provided by the policy. A close examination of a health care system will show exactly how the policy makers and their chief implementers view the patients/clients they serve, as well as the various categories of health personnel who provide the service. Let us take a few simple examples. Where is the health care facility situated? Can those for whom it is primarily designed reach it without great loss of time and at a reasonable cost? Can personnel reach it without severe financial outlay? Is the service available at times suited to the working person? These are only a few questions that can be raised, but they demonstrate concern for consumers and providers of health care.

Is the facility under-equipped, dirty and understaffed, both quanti-tatively and qualitatively? Does the system of managing the service, and particularly the system of managing the patient care aspect, demonstrate to patients/clients, and to health workers, that the management of the system is deeply concerned about the human dignity and well-being of patients and personnel?

One does not need words to communicate to the users of the facility that their human dignity is not rated very highly if the answers to the above questions are in the affirmative.

The recipients of this care feel it. I am preparing a series of studies on the psychosocial aspects of our care in both 'White' and 'Black' hospi-tals, and am deeply aware of the insensitivity of the system unless tempered by thinking, caring health care personnel. One has only to visit the out-patients department of a large hospital for White patients and see the bewilderment, the resignation, the feeling of helplessness of old-age pensioners and indigent persons who have no other recourse for health care to know what I am talking about.

Who meets the sick person at the front door of the hospital? And how are the admissions done? Have you noticed how the clerk, porter, or nurse aide calls out 'Van der Merwe' or 'Smith'? No 'Mrs' or 'Mr', just the nonentity 'Smith' or 'Van der Merwe'. Have you witnessed the impatient manner in which the aged, the confused, the weak and the helpless are treated? Is this not hurtful communication which disregards the human dignity and feelings of individuals? Have you witnessed the pathetic grati-tude of these people for a kind word, a helping hand, a friendly smile, the touch of a comforting hand? Why is this so? Insecure and unwell, they are at the mercy of the system, and the quality of organisation in the system communicates either security or insecurity. Quality communi-cation breaks down because it cannot stand up to the mechanics and dynamics of the system.

This happens in hospitals for Whites. It happens in equal measure in hospitals and clinics for Black patients, because our system of organisation does not facilitate meaningful communication. Have you ever witnessed the bewilderment of a tribal mother, an old grandmother or grandfather who not only fears the activities in the huge hospital or clinic complex, but has untold language and cultural barriers to surmount? Have you ever noticed how they are bullied and shunted around by insensitive porters and clerks, and how nurses and doctors grow impatient with them because they cannot obtain a coherent case history because of language difficulties? The attitude of health personnel, if not always their words, show that they have no time to waste – there is so much to do. Have you seen the total bewilderment of a tribal person or an aged individual who has no watch or who cannot read or write and who has received a multiple prescription with varying dosages and times for taking the medications? At best there are a few mumbled, hurried words of instruc-tion from an overworked nurse, words that the illiterate, culture-bound person does not comprehend. The system does not cater for such situ-ations. There is no time, and perhaps not enough money, to provide an effective service in this regard. Is it not surprising that the communication fails? The patient does not take the expensive medicine he is given, but returns to a traditional healer who understands what he is saying and communicates with him in terms he can understand, and with whom he has built up a relationship of trust. The core of good communication is trust.

I want to emphasise that the personnel are not unkind people. The system has failed to teach many how to handle human beings, and its management methods add to this failure. Frequently the patient numbers and the unsatisfactory ratio of personnel to patients aggravate the situation. In the rush of work and the confusion caused by cultural and language barriers, communication fails.

Communication for quality care is a matter as much for the attention of the system as it is for the individual health worker. Without adequate resources for the heavy patient load, communication cannot be effective. This inevitably affects the quality of health care and, *ipso facto*, of nursing care. The system must demonstrate its concern for the patient, for the community it serves, and for the health workers who serve it.

Indirect communication: the status the system assigns to the nursing service

Let me take another aspect of communication which undoubtedly affects the quality of nursing care. I refer to the subconscious relegation of the nursing service to a subservient position in the system. It is a form of communication which denigrates not only the nurses in the particular service, but the entire profession in that area. It is an unrecognised form of communication which will ultimately destroy the basis of quality nursing care, because nurses are no longer prepared to tolerate this and are protesting with their 'feet'. They are leaving nursing. I hasten to add that this does not apply everywhere.

I have identified eight key elements in this situation. You may recognise some of these elements. I assure you that they exist and they bedevil communications. They are the following:

   (i) Relegation of the most senior nurse manager in the system to a position subordinate to the most senior non-medical administrative officer.
  (ii) Withholding of information which is the just due of the nursing personnel on such issues as personnel policies, salaries, working conditions and the personal rights of the individual, as well as information about the specific goals of the organisation for each section of the service and for the organisation as a whole. There is a thick blanket of silence on issues which deeply affect the working life of the nurse and the quality of care she delivers.
 (iii) The manner is which the authorities in the system concerned view the role of the nurse *vis-à-vis* that of the doctor and other categories of health personnel. There are still authorities who view the role of the nurse as that of 'handmaiden' to the doctor and as general factotum.
  (iv) The workload that authorities expect nurses to carry and the extent to which they make it possible for nurses to provide innovative, creative and concerned nursing care.

(v) The unwillingness or the laggardness of many authorities to enable nursing personnel to keep abreast of developments in their profession through appropriate in-service education and, where necessary, appropriate formal education.

(vi) The lack of awareness that it is important to express appreciation for a job well done once in a while.

(vii) The lack of consultation with nursing personnel in order to meet new demands on the service, or to improve the quality of the existing service and the job satisfaction of personnel.

(viii) The disregard and even wilful denial by some authorities of the legitimate basic educational needs and rights of the nurse to enable her to take and maintain her rightful place as an effective member of the health team and as an educated member of society. Communication in this regard by both insensitive authorities and aggrieved nurses has done (and continues to do) nursing irreparable harm, placing it in an invidious position *vis-à-vis* other health professions.

I have selected these eight issues as examples of some types of communication which reflect deeply ingrained attitudes towards the true significance of the role of the nurse in the system. I have served the South African Nursing Association for 43 years, and throughout this time these eight issues have dominated discussions and negotiations. I regret to say that they are still with us, for as soon as they are eliminated in one area they arise in another. Biased attitudes and lack of knowledge of the role of nurses are important elements of this negative form of communication.

The position of the most senior nurse manager

Let me deal with another aspect of negative indirect communication within the system as it affects the nursing profession and its place within the system. One does not need words to describe the status assigned to a group. It is necessary only to consider the position of the most senior nurse manager in the group. Where is the most senior nurse manager's office situated? How does it compare with that of the most senior non-medical administrator? How does her salary compare with that of the most senior non-medical administrator? What role does the most senior nurse manager play in policy making, overall planning and daily overall management decisions?

Does the most senior nurse manager have the status and active role of one of the three top administrators in the health care facility? Does the top non-medical administrative officer ensure that copies of relevant material in *Government Gazettes*, circulars and directives from the central authority reach her? Is she the senior hostess of the service, or does she have to take a back seat to the wives of politicians, doctors and hospital administrators? Such recognition or non-recognition of her role proclaims loudly and clearly to all the personnel in the health care facility the standing of the nursing profession in that facility.

The question must be asked, however, whether the most senior nurse manager has been relegated to a subsidiary role, or has in fact relegated herself to this position because she is not equal to the task? Whatever the case it is a disastrous picture that is communicated to all personnel, particularly the nurses, as well as to the community.

These are not inconsequent statements. The positive or negative answers to these illustrate some of the forms of positive or negative communication within the health care hierarchy which assign a status and role to the nursing personnel. Negative aspects breed resentment and finally affect the quality of patient care.

The purpose of health care institutions – quality patient care

The purpose of our health care institutions is to ascertain and to meet the health care needs of our patients/clients and to fulfil the purpose of the legislature and our own roles in the prevention of ill-health, the promotion of good health and the healing and rehabilitation of the victims of illness and trauma. The quality of our patient care depends on what we communicate of our interest and intent, how we convey this concern through the quality of the management of the health care organisations, how we personalise the care of each individual, how we share our interest and concern with the patient/client and health workers, and how we help both the consumer and the provider of health care to fulfil their respective roles in a purposeful, humanistic manner.

Role recognition and fulfilment are powerful means of effective communication in the health care situation, as indeed they are in any occupation. The system creates problems because of its volume and complexity and tends to depersonalise both receivers and providers of care, for it tends to make a factory of the health care system.

The role of the nurse manager in nurturing positive communication for quality care

In looking at the question of communication and how it ultimately affects the quality of nursing care, I want to start with the nurse manager and work down to the ward/clinic situation. If the top nurse manager is equal to her task she will endeavour to straighten out her own role and equate it with those of others at the top management level of the health care facility. She will need the support of her professional association in this. Therefore I will bypass this aspect and look at her communication role in direct relationship with the nursing personnel.

The nurse manager is not only manager of the nursing service, she is the chief communicator in the nursing service. She delineates roles and interprets these to higher authority, to practitioners, to other health workers, to the community at large, and to would-be recruits to nursing. She is the key figure in the provision of quality care. Why do I say this? Let us look at what Jethro said to Moses more than 4 000 years ago, and ask ourselves: Is this not a perfect description of the roles of both manager and chief communicator? Does this not show that the quality of the service filters down from the manager, and that communication is its essence?

Jethro said to Moses:

Be though for the people to Godward, that thou mayest bring their causes unto God;

And thou shalt teach them ordinances and laws and the work they must do;

Moreover thou shalt provide out of all the people, able men, such as fear God, men of truth, hating covetousness, and place such over them, to be rulers of thousands, rulers of hundreds, rulers of fifties and rulers of ten;

And let them judge the people at all seasons, and it shall be that every great matter they shall bring unto thee, but every small matter they shall judge, so shall it be easier for thyself, and they shall bear in the burden with thee;
And if thou shall do this thing, and God commands thee so, then shalt thou be able to endure, and all the people shall also go to their place in peace (Exodus 18: 19-23).

Do not these verses state more clearly than any words of mine that communication is the very core of management control, that the nurse administrator must delegate authority to capable persons, that she herself must be the channel of communication between her service and higher authority, and that the quality of this communication will affect the well-being of those below her? Do not they clearly state that the nurse manager must be explicit in the formulation of rules, in providing guidelines, in ensuring that people know how to do their jobs and what is expected of them? Do not they show that she must delineate the scope of their authority, that she must choose persons of quality and ability who are not jealous of others to maintain the service, and that she must permit and require those under her to make decisions within the scope of their authority and responsibility, so that authority and responsibility become shaped?

Do not these verses also show that the value systems of the leader and of the sub-leaders influence the purpose and priorities of the system and direct the amount and nature of the effort needed to attain the purpose of the organisation? As far back as the days of Moses, competent leadership implied efficiency in the communication process as the basis of management.

The characteristics and ability of the nurse leader will determine the type of communication that will evolve. Will it be communication as 'power over people', or will it be communication as 'power with people'? The quality of management in nursing is dependent on the latter.

We are all aware that it is the primary function of the chief nurse manager to:

(i) define nursing policy, its purpose and objectives
(ii) identify and describe standards for quality nursing care
(iii) devise an organisational system, delineate roles and assign responsibilities
(iv) identify criteria and methods for ensuring quality control
(v) devise a system of creative supervision and evaluation of personnel
(vi) devise a system for ensuring competence and the maintenance of a sound philosophy of nursing
(vii) ensure that every member of the nursing team knows exactly what is expected of her, how she will be evaluated and what sort of help she may expect to improve her performance.

We are all aware that the philosophy of quality care emanates from the top. It is a philosophy that is caught, not taught.

All of the above relate specifically to communication between nurse managers and personnel. I do not wish to focus on them, but on some other aspects of communication emanating from the nurse administrator.

The nurse administrator must ensure that communication is effective

A fundamental function of the nurse administrator is to ensure that communication is clear, direct and takes into consideration not only policy and objectives, but personnel ability and human dignity, and that this is the case at all levels of the nursing service. On this rests the smooth functioning of the organisation and the ultimate well-being of patients and staff.

It is the nurse administrator's primary duty to create a personnel climate conducive to the accurate and free flow of information. To do this she must ensure that the nursing personnel not only understand all the dimensions of their respective jobs, but also acquire a basic understanding of communication concepts and the implications of these for every-day relationships and care of patients. Communication effectiveness is a key issue in nursing service. The nurse administrator needs a constant interchange of communication and to gather accurate facts, for without these she cannot make wise decisions. In assessing the level of communication necessary for smooth administration, the maintenance of morale or quality care, she has to assess the quality of interpersonal relationships in the nursing service, for wastage of personnel and poor quality care have their roots in poor interpersonal relationships.

For effective management the nurse administrator has to look at the methods and channels of communication and the accuracy and completeness of information. She has to bear in mind that emotion is involved in all communications. Meaning is also conveyed by what is *not* said – by attitudes and expressions, body movements and tone of voice.

It is her task to ensure that no obstacles lie in the way of staff communication, that she listens to and thinks about what the staff says, and that she tries to determine their real opinions.

It is the task of the nurse manager to ensure a free flow of communication and to coach her personnel in effective means of communication. The more effective the leader's communication, the more effective her leadership and the performance of her personnel will be. The leader who ensures identification and acknowledgement of individual abilities within the group and of group strengths enhances the contribution of her service. Interdependent, collaborative efforts by the group cemented by sound communication techniques facilitate the accomplishment of goals, while threats and non-recognition of individual and group performance inhibit quality care.

There is a need to evolve group discussions with her personnel in a non-threatening, safe environment. Only through discussion can she set realistic, attainable objectives and arrive at mutual understanding of problems and goals. Only by unbiased discussion with due concern for the contribution of all can she hope to obtain commitment from each member of the group. In directing a service there are six problems she must guard against, namely:

(i) communication overloads
(ii) communication starvation

(iii) incorrect communication
(iv) communication malfunctions
 (v) the misuse of communication
(vi) lack of reinforcement and feedback.

If she disregards these essential factors in communication she will not ensure quality care, but will cause chaos, resentment and high personnel turnover.

Communication and the charge nurse

Jethro was quite right when he emphasised the need to select the right persons to act as group or sectional leaders. I believe one should not appoint a nurse to a chargeship position unless she truly understands the philosophy of nursing. She cannot be an effective leader, care giver or teacher if she does not understand that the very act of nursing is communication of a special kind. She must understand that it is fundamentally a form of communication of one's concern for one's fellow men, and that in carrying out the acts of nursing there is a rich communication amalgam of all the empirical and scientific knowledge that has been developed and communicated to nursing from the earliest period of man's existence to the present day. The communication process is a rich mix of philosophy, concern and conversion of knowledge into action. She must understand that it is the dominant aspect of our practice. How we interpret our role as nurses communicates what we believe we are and determines the quality of our actions.

Nursing's foundations rest on interpersonal relationships with patients/clients, relatives, the community, other team members and employers. The quality of interpersonal relationships determines the quality of care.

So frequently we forget that the personnel and patient climate in the ward/department or clinic is dependent on the person-in-charge of that unit. Human relations can be completely ruined by the attitude of the person-in-charge. She does not have to say an angry word – the way she looks, her gestures, the way she walks and her tone of voice can all arouse fear and tension in personnel and patients. The manner in which she fulfils her role constitutes a most powerful form of communication. Her dress, attitude, confidence, approachability, empathy and sympathy; her ability to act as a source person; her ability to remain cool and decisive in a crisis; her charm, friendliness and innate courtesy; and her helpfulness communicate a relationship of trust. Patients feel safe with a person who represents their image of the competent, kind nurse. Young students see in such a nurse the personification of their ideal. They want to be like her.

Cooperation at every level is a firm foundation for the communication process. A cooperative attitude is essential for sound interpersonal relationships and quality patient care. Creative thinking which leads to the identification of correct facts and thinking about these facts before taking action is fundamental for sound communication. The choice of the right word to the right person at the right time in the right place and in the right manner comes from careful thinking and the wise use of the art of communication. It is constructive and creative, not a blocking process.

Last, the way in which the nurse practitioner in charge of a unit interprets the dependent, interdependent and independent functions of the
nurse to her personnel and to students, as well as to doctors and other
health care personnel, will help to ensure that registered nurse practitioners will be law-abiding and fully aware:

   (i) that they are totally dependent on the law for their right to practise
      and how they exercise this right

  (ii) that they have a joint personal and professional responsibility with
      the doctor for the care of their patients and a duty to be cooperative
      in the interests of good patient care, as befits a responsible pro-
      fessional colleague

 (iii) that they are independent professional practitioners, personally
      accountable for their dependent, interdependent and independent
      functions, acts and omissions. On accountability rests the quality of
      nursing care. It is a factor that must be communicated to student
      nurses constantly and must be engraved on the hearts and minds
      of all nurse practitioners, for accountability for the quality of nurs-
      ing care is part of the system of acceptance of public trust which is
      the hallmark of the professional person. It is evidence of the self-
      discipline that a profession requires of its members, for it is evidence
      of the values, attitudes, and knowledge of nurses towards their right
      and responsibility to provide quality care. It is part of the credibility
      of the nursing profession. The foundation for all this is a firm
      knowledge base and the will, ability and sense of responsibility to
      transfer this knowledge to the treatment and care of human beings
      in need of nursing care.

Finally, let us try to communicate to our nurses the gift of enthusiasm
for concern, action and cooperation, and for accountability. If we have
helped each one to think about these issues, if we have helped them to
implement these concepts, we have 'shared' and we have communicated
in the truest sense of the word. We will have made our contribution to
quality nursing care.

Bibliography

Alexander, EL. 1978. *Nursing Administration in the hospital and health care system.*
   2nd ed. Saint Louis: CV Mosby. (Chapter 11.)

Arndt, C & Huckabey, LM. 1980. *Nursing administration.* 2nd ed. Saint Louis: CV
   Mosby. (p 265.)

Casson, HN. No date. *How to get things done.* London: The Efficiency House
   Magazine.

Deegan, AX. 19??. *Coaching − a management skill for improving individual perform-*
   ance. Reading: Addison Wesley Publishing Co. (Chapter 2.)

Divencenti, M. 1977. *Administering nursing service.* 2nd ed. Boston: Little Brown
   & Co. (pp 278-287.)

Fenlason, AE. 1962. *Essentials of interviewing.* New York: Harper & Row.

Kron, T. 1966. *Nursing team leadership.* Philadelphia: WB Saunders (pp 43-49.)

Kron, T. 1972. *Communication in Nursing.* 2nd ed. Philadephia: WB Saunders & Co.

Lemin, B. 1977. *First line nursing management.* Tunbridge Wells: Pitman Medical
   Publishing Co. (Chapter 12.)

Ley, P & Spelman, MS. 1967. *Communication with the patient.* London: The Staples
   Press.

Marram, GD. 1973. *The group approach in nursing practice.* Saint Louis: CV Mosby.
   (Chapter 6.)

McFarlane, J & Castledine, G. 1982. *A guide to the Practice of Nursing using the Nurs-*
   ing Process. London: CV Mosby.

Moloney, MM. 1979. *Leadership in Nursing.* Saint Louis: CV Mosby. (Chapter 4.)

Stevens, BJ. 1978. *The Nurse as Executive.* Wakefield: Contemporary Publishing Inc. (Chapter 5.)

Travelbee, J. 1966. *Interpersonal aspects of Nursing.* Philadelphia: TA Davis Co. (Chapter 8.)

Overview of the practice issues relevant to the development of the ethos of nursing

Four major issues are discussed in this section. They are presented because they are causing major concern to the profession, and because they are problems which arise in all countries. They are of particular concern to the 97 national nurses' associations which are in membership with the International Council of Nurses.

It is a sad commentary on the 'state of the art' that these issues should be so widespread. The following questions may be asked:

(i) Have nurses attempted to identify the causal factors which give rise to these issues?

(ii) Do nurses have sufficient assertiveness to rectify these problems?

(iii) Are not the nurses who are most vocal about the lack of a positive image of nursing and prone to burnout, those who have poor images of themselves as people and hence as nurses? Is not this harping on the poor image of the nurse done by nurses who are content to be doctors' 'handmaidens' rather than their professional colleagues? As one medical specialist said:

> We would never have dared to treat a certain nurse as a handmaiden, she was our valued colleague who contributed to our success as healers. We could discuss the patients with her, we took her advice and we would never have dared to look on her as a subordinate. Even if we were foolish enough to wish to do so, she would have let us know in no uncertain terms that she was our partner and not our servant. She would have done so without being discourteous but we would have known exactly what our role relationships were. The way she practised her profession, and not words, made her our partner.

(iv) Is not the poor dress sense some nurses show in the way that they wear their 'uniform' (protective clothing) due to the fact that their professional socialisation did not include issues such as deportment, the correct wearing of uniforms (protective clothing), public speaking and the social graces required of a hostess to the public and peers?

(v) Do nurses lack the type of leadership locally, regionally and nationally that could eliminate some of the more blatant problems?

(vi) Could not nurses tackle some of the problems through in-service education programmes?

Poor communication in the nursing profession is a problem which urgently requires attention. It is *the* most clamant problem facing the profession. The ethos of nursing as perceived by other professions, many members of the profession and some members of the public reflects this shortcoming.

The nursing profession must improve the quality of its communication, for good communication forms the basis of not only high quality nursing practice, but also of the image projected by the profession. The issue of communication has been with nurses in this country since the beginnings of professional nursing. In 1991 nurses will celebrate 100 years of state registration. How will we judge this issue when preparing our centenary celebrations, and how will the profession be judged in the year 2000?

PART

4

The regulation of nursing

9

Some thoughts on the Nursing Act
(Act 50 of 1978)

[A 1986 South African perspective]

Introductory commentary

The question of the relevance of the Nursing Act to contemporary development of the health services and of the nursing profession is raised repeatedly.

This address attempts to deal with this question by highlighting the purpose of the Act, the mechanisms for implementing the purpose of the Act, and the significance of the provisions for the citizen and the nurse. It demonstrates how the legislation enacted by a country inevitably exercises a major influence on the development of the nursing ethos in that country.

THE ADDRESS

Introduction

The Nursing Act 50 of 1978 is currently the most advanced nurse practice Act in the world. It has enabled the nursing profession in South Africa to reach the zenith of professional development, the essence of which is control of the profession by the profession under Act of Parliament in the interests of the public good. A dual benefit arises from such an Act. The legislature ensures that the profession is entrusted with the public good, but in so doing it also gives the profession special recognition and status in that it is seen to be competent and responsible enough to carry out such a trust and to be willing to accept this trust and to be held accountable for its stewardship.

South Africa has always been and, we trust, will remain, a world leader in respect of nursing legislation. Although we hold such an enviable position, one wonders whether all members of the profession in South Africa have a good general knowledge of the provisions of the Act? Do all nurses know what the purpose of the Act is? Do they realise that every action carried out by the South African Nursing Council under the authority of the Act enhances in some manner the safety of the nursing care received by the public? At the same time, it also enhances the standing, the knowledge and the ethical norms of the profession. Similarly, every positive action taken by the Nursing Association to enhance the knowledge, skills, integrity and socio-economic status of the profession is ultimately beneficial to the public as well.

The availability of a competent, knowledgeable, law-abiding, ethically conforming nursing force is part of the human capital of a country. It is part of its riches. It helps to contribute to the public good while enhancing the image and status of the profession.

Overall purpose of the Nursing Act not recognised

It appears that the overall purpose of the Nursing Act is not recognised. There is a tendency to restrict views about the Act to the list of functions of the two statutory bodies that are established under the provisions of the Act.

Superficially, the powers of the two statutory bodies appear to be diametrically opposed: one appears to protect the public, and the other the nurse. Yet there is inevitably a convergence of purpose in that both of the statutory bodies ultimately serve the public good, irrespective of the manner in which this can be done. Ironically, both bodies may interpret their responsibilities in a way that may harm the public good and may exercise their powers in a way that is detrimental to the public good. In such a situation Parliament, which entrusted them with the powers to govern or to represent their profession, as the case may be, will have no other recourse but to withdraw the powers entrusted to the profession. Control of the profession would then pass into the hands of the bureaucratic machine, and representation of the profession's interests would pass to a variety of diverse non-professional organisations.

The ultimate purpose of South Africa's Nurse Practice Act, the Nursing Act, is to serve the public good, for this is what nursing is all about.

The South African Nursing Council the standard setting and control body

The South African Nursing Council is the body charged under the Act with the approval of the education and training of nurses – at both the basic and the advanced levels; the registration or enrolment of all who practise nursing; prescribing the scope of practice of the nurse; and the disciplinary control of the profession. This is all primarily in the interests of the public good, but in the end also benefits the profession.

Let us take a brief look at each of these functions and see how each one safeguards the interests of the public and enhances the interests of the nurse. This latter aspect is generally forgotten when the role and functions of the South African Nursing Council are taught.

Control of education and training

Section 15 of the Nursing Act provides for control over the education and training of nurses by the South African Nursing Council. This section specifically states:

> notwithstanding anything to the contrary in any law contained, no person or institution may offer or provide any education or training which is intended to qualify any person to practise the profession of nursing or midwifery to which the provisions of this Act apply, unless such education and training have been approved by the Council (Section 15(1)).

This means that all formal courses of education and training leading to a qualification must be approved by the Council. Private hospitals must take note of this provision. It does not matter whether a course is offered by a university, a small hospital or an occupational health nursing school – if it is intended to qualify the nurse for some nursing activity, it must be approved by the Council. Approval of training such as in-service education courses which do not result in certification does not fall under the provisions of the Act.

Section 15(2) provides that institutions wishing to offer any form of education and training must apply to the Council for approval, presenting to it full particulars of the proposed programme.

Section 15(5) clearly states that it is an offence, that is a criminal offence, to provide any education and training if Council has not approved it. The penalties for proved transgression of this proviso are very heavy, being R500 or imprisonment for six months, or both. Please note that it is a police matter and the courts take the action necessary. It is interesting to note that on being found guilty by the courts registered nurses (midwives) who have been involved in such an activity may have to face a disciplinary action by the South African Nursing Council. Establishment of guilt by a court, irrespective of the sentence meted out by the court, constitutes *prima facie* evidence of misconduct by the nurse and the Council must take action.

There is a need for strict control of the education and training of nurses. First, the public must be protected against unscrupulous persons who provide inadequate or unsuitable education and training programmes which will inevitably harm the public. Second, there is a need to protect the person (the nurse) who is misled by such unscrupulous persons and who will find on completion of the course that the qualification is worthless.

Control of the education and training of nurses ensures that the persons who are registered or enrolled have achieved a definite level of education aimed at meeting the nursing care needs of the country. The public safety is potentially ensured in that the holder of an approved qualification is entitled to a certain scope of practice, has obtained at least the minimum standard of education and training to enable her to practise within the parameters of the prescribed scope of practice and has the necessary foundation for further professional education.

At the same time the status of the profession is safeguarded because its members must meet certain educational requirements which are nationally recognised, which measure up to the education of other professionals at a similar level and which enjoy a measure of international recognition. Such an educational qualification is a valuable possession. The act of protecting the public has a reciprocal benefit for the profession.

Registration and enrolment

The act of registration or enrolment implies three things which are of vital importance to the public, namely:

(i) proof of having completed an approved programme of education and training within the parameters of the particular category of nursing practice

(ii) proof of a minimal level of knowledge and skill to carry out the prescribed scope of practice

(iii) proof of the fact that the nurse is willing and able to be accountable for her own acts of omission and commission and by registration or enrolment automatically submits herself to the disciplinary control of her profession.

Any person from outside the borders of South Africa who does not comply with the minimum educational and training requirements pertaining to South African programmes must make up defects in training prior to registration. Utilising the services of such persons in the capacity of either registered or enrolled persons is a criminal offence. If such a person wants to work until full registration is possible she may seek enrolment either as an enrolled nurse or as an enrolled nursing assistant, or may obtain restricted registration for a period not exceeding two years under the provisions of Section 21.

Registration and enrolment standards protect the profession as well as the public, for while ensuring the public good through the three important dimensions of registration and enrolment, they also enhance the status and the standing of the profession in that the nurse is entitled to use certain letters after her name, they give entry to certain levels of appointment, they confer a definite scope of practice on a nurse, they open certain doors for further education and they give the nurse a recognised and important social identity. Today registration in particular is regarded as the 'cachet of professionalism' worldwide.

The protection of the public against imposters, or against nurses whose registration or enrolment has lapsed, is ensured by Section 27 of the Act, which makes practice by persons who are not registered an offence with which the courts will deal. While such protection of the public is vitally important and is the primary reason for Section 27, there is no doubt that the section also acts as a protective mechanism for the law-abiding members of the nursing profession. The status of the registered or enrolled person is jealously guarded primarily in the interests of the public, but also because it enhances the status of the profession.

Scope of practice

The scope of practice of nurses and midwives is defined by a regulation promulgated under Section 45(q) of the Act. This is a most significant proviso, for it unambiguously indicates that the Council, and only the Council, can say what the scope of practice of the nurse is, for this must be related to the basic education and training which the Council controls. Defining the scope of practice is in the public interest and in the interests of other health professionals who make up the health team, but it is also of vital importance to the status of the profession and to the individual practice of the nurse, who is clearly designated a practitioner in her own right. There is without doubt a reciprocal benefit to the public and the profession.

Disciplinary control

Disciplinary control of the profession is one of the most important functions of the Council, for it is aimed at ensuring orderly and ethical practice in nursing. It is intended primarily as protection for the public, so that the public may be safe in the hands of nurses and the trust between the profession and the public may be maintained. However, it is significant that the good name of the profession looms large in the Act. Section 29(1) refers to 'improper or disgraceful conduct, or conduct which, when regard is had to such person's profession, is improper or disgraceful'. It is inevitable that disciplinary control benefits both public and profession, for a profession which maintains high ethical standards which are jealously guarded by its Council receives due recognition for this in the form of recognition of its standing and of its professionhood.

Disciplinary control is a most serious matter. This is recognised in the provisions of the Act, which ensure that disciplinary action shall be taken according to the principles of law, with justice for all and malice towards none.

This brief overview of the functions of the Council indicates that it is inaccurate to say, as we so often do, that 'the Council is there to protect the interests of the public, and the Association is there to protect the interests of the nurse'. I believe that this is a half-truth, for each function of protection of the public also indirectly or directly confers a certain status on the nursing profession and the development of the profession is in the interests of the public.

It can be argued that such enhancement of the status demands greater accountability from the profession in the interests of the public, but whichever way we look at it the functions of the Council which are designed to protect the public at the same time confer a certain privileged status on the profession, so we may quite rightly say that the Council enhances the interests of the profession without necessarily protecting them. I became very much aware of this feature of our Act when I studied the nurse practice Acts of some other countries.

The objectives of the Council

The objectives of the Council confer on the nursing profession in South Africa a role and status which so far appears to be unique in the world. When acting within its stated objectives the Council not only serves the public at the highest level, but acts in a special consultative capacity to the Minister under whose jurisdiction the Nursing Act is implemented. Parliament has realised that the nursing profession has a major contribution to make to the delivery of health services and values this contribution. It has given nurses the right to make their representations at any time, and to do so on any matter affecting the health of the nation and the practice of their profession. In so doing it has acknowledged the special expertise and status of the profession. This enhances the prestige of the profession while serving the public good.

The South African Nursing Association

The Act provides for a statutory professional association of nurses to which all practising nurses have to belong. When this proviso (Section 38) was incorporated into the Nursing Act, Parliament aimed at canalising nursing aspirations and efforts into constructive channels which, while recognising and striving for the legitimate socio-economic improvements of the profession, would secure the desired changes by professional negotiation, remembering at all times that the profession of nursing exists only by reason of the needs of health services and the sick (Searle 1965:233).

While the daily activities of the Association concern the socio-economic development of the profession, the end product of this activity is the well-being of the public through the development of the profession, research and the representation of the interests of the members. The converging point for the Council and the Association is the public welfare, although this is attained in different ways. The Council ensures public well-being and contributes to the development of the profession by the manner in which peer group control is exercised, while the Association performs the same function by developing opportunities for socio-economic development and for the professional growth and development of individuals who will practise nursing as responsible and fully accountable practitioners abiding by the standards and ethical values enunciated by the South African Nursing Council.

The special role of the Association

I believe that the Association has a special role as the mouthpiece of the profession:

(i) to bring educational needs to the notice of the Council and to other relevant authorities

(ii) to develop among its members the ability to serve the profession as experts of various aspects of nursing and nursing education

(iii) to develop among its members the ability to take part in the peer group control of the profession by serving on the Council, not as representatives of the electorate, but as expert servants of the public. This is a most important duty of the Association, for in reality it is the 'King maker', the body from whom the majority of the members of the Council are drawn.

The Association is the profession and the profession is the Association, and from its ranks the persons who will control the standards of the profession during their term of office must be drawn.

There is mutual interdependence between Council and Association, even if at times this is only nebulous. The control of the profession can only be as good as the Association is able to make it. In the years that lie ahead let us give attention to the overall meaning of the nursing Act, which embraces the public good as well as the good of the profession, and let us be truly professional in the way in which we view the meaning of the Nursing Act, for through the professionhood of the individual will the professionalism of nursing be given meaning.

References

Searle, C. 1965. *The history of the development of Nursing in South Africa 1652-1960.* Cape Town: Struik.

10

The International Council of Nurses

examines 'The Regulation of Nursing' 1986

[Important issues in the report on the Regulation of
Nursing (ICN)]

ADDRESS 1987

In 1985 the International Council of Nurses (ICN) presented a report on
'The Regulation of Nursing' as a report on 'The Present, a position for
the Future'. The report was based on a project conducted by Margareta
M Styles for the Professional Services Committee of that organisation and
was accepted by the Council of National Representatives as a position
paper.

The aim of the project was to collect, organise and report on data pertaining to the regulatory systems current in nursing and to devise guidelines regarding the official position that the ICN should take to assist its
member associations to evaluate and develop their systems.

The overall finding was that throughout the world (South Africa, not
being a member of the ICN, was not included in the study) the regulation
of nursing is:

ill-defined and diverse, educational requirements and legal definitions of nursing
are generally inadequate for the complexity and expansion of the nursing role
as it is emerging in response to health care needs; and the goals and standards
of the profession are less apparent than one half century ago (ICN Report
1983:3).

The report deals with aspects such as the approach to the study of occupational regulation; a historical overview; the present situation worldwide;
an analysis of issues such as definitions of regulatory terminology, occupational terminology and structure; the philosophy, purpose and politics
of regulation; the economics of regulation; the scope of practice; standards of regulation; characteristics of the regulatory processes; nursing
in transition; and the ICN position.

Analysis of the issues

Analysis of the issues indicates that the regulation of nursing practitioners
takes place by means of two systems of control, namely *practice* and *title*
control. In South Africa we refer to practice and title control as *mandatory*
control, both the practice of nursing and the title 'nurse' being protected.
In some countries only the title 'nurse' is protected, anyone being permitted to perform nursing acts.

Licensure or registration is a mechanism of government control which may or may not be exercised through peer group control, as is the case in South Africa.

Certification is not a government issue. Credentialing is a generic term for all regulatory mechanisms, state and/or professional.

Titles are not comparable in the various countries.

An important issue highlighted by the report is whether nursing is distinctive from, subsidiary to, preparatory to or integrative with other occupations. All four of these positions are present in nursing regulation systems.

(i) Nursing is *distinctive* or *autonomous* when it is by law *accountable to the public* and when all career advancement is possible *within* the profession itself. *This is the position in South Africa.*

(ii) Nursing is *subsidiary* or *externally controlled* when nurses are required by law to report all their actions to doctors who 'take responsibility for them' and where nursing schools are headed by doctors. *This is not the case in South Africa.*

(iii) Nursing is *preparatory* when by law nurses progress into careers in other health professions such as medicine or the supplementary health service professions. This is also not the case in South Africa.

(iv) Nursing is *integrative* when government job classifications provide for interchangeability with persons prepared in other fields.

The South African standpoint has always coincided with that of the World Health Organisation (WHO), which states:

Nursing practice needs to be autonomous and accountable and legislation that embodies unrealistic restrictions should be re-examined and changes instituted. Nursing care is complementary to all other types of care, but it makes its own unique contribution to health services as a whole (WHO 1982:32).

The report states:

If the nursing profession as a whole agrees
(1) that its members should be prepared for the development of their greatest potential as citizens and for the achievement of the highest objectives of nursing care,
(2) that it will be fully accountable for its actions and refuses to be confined to a lower standard or a lesser social contribution, and
(3) that is deserves to be properly recognised for this contribution,
then this commitment should set the goals for professional regulation around the world (ICN Report 1986:32).

The report endorses a stand taken by the ICN in 1969 that:

It is the duty of the nursing profession of every country to work for suitable legislature enactment regulating the education of nurses and protection of the interests of the public by securing state examination and public registration with the proper penalties for not enforcing same (ICN 1969:4 as quoted in ICN Report 1986:32).

The ICN's stand is simply that 'Nursing legislation should include provision for control of nursing education, licensing/registration, and practice (ICN 1969 as quoted in ICN Report 1986:32).

A further significant statement quoted in the report is taken from the ICN Principles. This states that:

> the purpose of professional licensure is, on the one hand, to secure to society the benefits which come from the services of a highly skilled group and, on the other hand, to protect society from those who are not highly skilled yet profess to be, or from those who, being highly skilled, are nevertheless so unprincipled as to misuse their superior knowledge to the disadvantage of the people.
>
> Regulation of a profession or a vocation must primarily protect the public health, safety, welfare or morals by prohibiting practice in a field in which incompetent practice would create a threat to the public, and it must tend to ensure competency by requiring persons who engage in those professions to qualify themselves under standards established by the state (ICN 1969:9 as quoted in ICN Report 1986:32).

The ICN has consistently stated that unauthorised persons should be prevented from practising nursing. This is supported by the International Labour Organisation (ILO) in its statement that specifies that legislation should 'limit the practice of the profession to duly authorised persons' (ILO 1982:1149). In other words, compulsory registration of all who practise nursing is advocated.

The question of the 'most competent, accessible, cost-effective health services' (ICN Report 1986:32) is addressed. In its pursuit of the goal 'Health for All by the year 2000', WHO (1982:29) states unequivocally:

> Nursing, among all the health professions, has the greatest potential for ensuring cost-effectiveness. Nurses are represented in any form of health service and since they work closely with patients they are in a position to assess the effects of the care rendered. Their voice needs to be heard in the debate on cost-effectiveness.

The report endorses this standpoint.

The report addresses the question of the scope of practice and refers to the desirability of promulgating regulations that are general so as to allow the nurse autonomy and scope for extending her functions.

Considerable discussion of the problems of the transition of nursing, of the need for change in some countries and of the right of nurses to speak for themselves is reflected in the report.

The ICN has taken a certain position regarding the regulation of nursing, namely that it should:

  (i) have an explicit purpose

  (ii) be drafted to fulfil its purpose

  (iii) have clear definitions of professional scope and accountability

  (iv) promote the fullest development of the profession in accordance with its social contribution

  (v) recognise the legitimate roles of the public, profession, government, employers and other professions in standard setting

  (vi) provide for representational balance

  (vii) be flexible so as to achieve objectives

(viii) observe the principle of universality within the parameters of professional identity and mobility, with due regard for local needs and circumstances

(xi) be honest and fair to all concerned

(x) recognise the equality and interdependence of professions.

The value of this report is inestimable. Margareta Styles has done a magnificent job, showing rare insight into the professional constraints and dilemmas in nursing worldwide. The ICN's stand sets the seal on the thoughts enunciated and the facts identified.

South African nurses should study this chapter in conjunction with the previous one so that they may judge whether nursing legislation in this country meets the criteria identified in the report.

The claim that the Nursing Act (and its regulations) is at present the most advanced nurse practice Act in the world is substantiated in this brief outline of the features which should characterise the regulation of nursing.

References

ICN. 1986. *The Regulation of Nursing*. Report. Geneva: ICN.
ILO. 1982. *International Labour Conventions and Recommendations*. Geneva: ILO.
WHO. 1982. *Nursing in support of the goal of health for all by the year 2000*. Geneva: WHO.

PART 5

Health for all by the year 2000

11

Constraints on the pursuit of the goal 'Health for all by the year 2000'

Introductory commentary

In Southern Africa professional and enrolled nurses are in the vanguard of the provision of health care. Wherever other health professionals are not available nurses provide the service necessary to the best of their ability.

The nursing profession is particularly concerned with the implementation of WHO's concept 'Health for all by the year 2000'. However, nurses must be aware of the many constraints on the pursuit of this goal. The health professions cannot work this miracle on their own, for health is not achieved in isolation. It is dependent on numerous economic, social, cultural, institutional and educational factors. There can be no health unless health problems are tackled on an intersectoral basis, with services such as agriculture, animal husbandry, water affairs and sanitation control, employment provisions, income-generating activities, housing, recreation, schooling, social development, family planning and family and community involvement all interacting in the social development of a community or nation. Health care provision forms only a part of this.

The constitution of the World Health Organisation (WHO) characterises health as a basic human right. The pronouncements and the policies of this organisation make it clear that the individual must exercise control over this right by means of his lifestyle, his care for his own health and that of his family, and his involvement in community work aimed at providing health care, preventing disease and bringing about social development.

Primary health care programmes must constitute the main thrust of the provision of health care. It cannot be over-emphasised that:

Primary health care is essential health care based on practical, scientifically sound and socially acceptable methods and technology made universally accessible to individuals and families in the community through their full participation and at a cost that the community and the country can afford to maintain at every stage of their development in the spirit of self-reliance and self-determination. It forms an integral part both of the country's health system, of which it is the central function and main focus, and of the overall social and economic development of the community. It is the first level of contact of individuals, the family and community with the national health system bringing health care as close as possible to where people live and work, and constitutes the first element of a continuing health care process (WHO & UNICEF 1978:4).

Primary health care requires political will, health professional commitment and community involvement to translate it into reality.

The majority of doctors and nurses do not know what community development means, or claim that they are too busy to become involved in it. The constraints listed in the address are all social indicators, the impact of which must

86

be blunted if social development is to take place. The effective introduction of primary health care is undermined by lack of knowledge on the methods of social development, identifying the strengths and weaknesses of a community, identifying leadership potential, motivating individuals and families to become involved, providing guidance on how to deal with health problems and the strengths, weaknesses and methods of communication.

Appropriate education of administrative personnel, health personnel and the communities to be served is essential for the effective implementation of a health service. Equally important is the education of personnel in all sectors of government, parastatal and private social development services. Far more attention must be given to the education of health personnel to ensure that they focus on individuals, families and the community and that they strive for inter-sectoral cooperation at all levels.

Primary health care provision has changed the role of the nurse dramatically, particularly that of Black and Coloured nurses, who are the main providers of such services. How effective is their inter-sectoral cooperation? Do they use the family as the focus in their health educational activities and when motivating community members to become involved in community health care and social development activities? How do they communicate with people requiring health care, and with those who must be persuaded to become involved in their own care or that of their families and the community?

How effective members of the nursing profession have been as social developers, health care providers, supervisors, advisers and resource persons will be seen in the year 2000 when an evaluation of the nation's state of health is made to see whether the goal of 'health for all' has been achieved. Not only the nursing profession, but all forms of social administration and the people themselves will be judged. It is hoped that they will not be found wanting!

Health professionals must develop the knowledge and skills to meet the objective in its full sense, that is health inclusive of social development. They must provide leadership through knowledge and with the will to achieve the goal. An assessment of the constraints on reaching the goal illustrates the magnitude of the problem and the knowledge and skills required by health professionals, social planners and administrators if they are to make any impact on these problems. What will the report be like in the year 2000?

THE ADDRESS

Introduction

The ideal of 'health for all by the year 2000' is evidently not an easy one to attain. As the century draws to a close there is mounting evidence that the numerous factors which militate against the attainment of health for all are in no way decreasing. Rather, their impact is being accentuated to the extent that there has been a comparative failure around the world to improve health indices, probably due to failure to understand the personal and social determinants of health and disease, but probably also to the lack of means to achieve an impact on the health indices. Lack of understanding and of 'know-how' is an important factor, but lack of the 'wherewithal' to achieve any measure of success is critical.

Factors which compound the problems and retard the development of an effective level of health for all are the following:

(i) The continuing high rate of population growth in underdeveloped communities. Some underdeveloped countries are beginning to succeed in their efforts to slow down the rate of population growth, but all underdeveloped countries should try to do so.

(ii) Progressive massive unemployment, not only because of:
- the flooding of the labour markets of the world by the young people produced by population explosions
- the retarded economic development of third world countries and the political instability of many of these countries

but also because of the worldwide slowing down of economic growth since the eighties. What the spin-offs will be for the underdeveloped countries when a resurgence in the economies of the developed countries occurs cannot be predicted with any degree of accuracy.

(iii) The progressive lowering of the nutritional level of the bulk of the world's population.

(iv) The decreasing amount of land available and incorrect utilisation of such land for food production.

(v) The accelerated rural-urban drift, which is leading to highly dangerous rates of urbanisation worldwide and the concomitant social, health and political problems. These are emerging on a mass scale in all the major cities and towns of the world. Reversal of this urban drift by development of the rural areas is a priority in all the countries of the world.

(vi) Very slow progress is being made in reducing illiteracy in the underdeveloped parts of the world. In the majority of underdeveloped countries a very significant proportion of children still do not attend primary school.

(vii) The inequitable distribution of the benefits of economic growth when this actually takes place, which results in a widening of the health gap in the underdeveloped countries.

(viii) The status of women in underdeveloped countries. Although a considerable amount of lip-service is being paid to this issue, virtually nothing is being done about it.

(ix) The mounting poverty that is 'the lot of substantial parts of the population of the Third World . . . It is of course this continuing poverty that is at the root of world's most pressing health problems' (WHO Sixth Report 1980:2). There is evidence that a number of developing countries are managing to reduce their overall levels of poverty and to improve their health indices, despite the fact that their per capita income levels are no more favourable than those of other countries in the region with poor health indices and similar poverty levels.

(x) The need for all nations to study the relationship between man and his environment. Much attention has been given to the oil crisis of 1973 and its effects on the economy and the social tensions of the world. In addition, increased pollution of the environment, the disastrous effects of progressive soil erosion and the steady increase in desert areas in the third world, particularly Africa, urgently require the attention of the governments of the affected regions.

(xi) While there is a decline in mortality rates in many countries, this is not universal, and the causes of death have not altered significantly in the third world.

> The most striking fact about mortality today is that despite the massive economic growth and technological progress of the period following the Second World War, the same basic complex of infectious, parasitic and respiratory diseases, compounded by nutritional deficiencies, still accounts for most of the world's deaths (WHO Sixth Report 1980:2).

Three decades of concerted effort by WHO and the governments of the third world have not managed to change this picture, which is characteristic of causes of death in underdeveloped countries. Yet the effort continues and it is hoped that by the end of this century preventable diseases will have a low incidence in third world countries.

(xii) The lack of reliable data on health issues. Data on morbidity and mortality profiles are not reliable due to inaccurate or frequently non-existent health statistics in many developing countries.

(xiii) Mounting evidence that certain communicable diseases, for example schistosomiasis and malaria, are on the increase or are resurging as major health problems. Little progress can be reported with regard to the control of tuberculosis and the sexually transmitted diseases. It appears that smallpox has been controlled, although there can never be certainty about this.

(xiv) Evidence that cardiovascular disease and cancer continue to be the greatest problem diseases in industrialised societies and that these conditions are on the increase in the middle-income countries.

(xv) The absence of high level health planning in all countries.

> Health planning has tended in many places to be a sporadic activity, carried out without recourse to experienced social and economic planners. The domination of the health planning process by members of the medical profession, sometimes to the exclusion of others, has not been helpful (WHO Sixth Report I 1980:3).

(xvi) The urgent need to find solutions to the many outstanding problems experienced in health manpower planning, training and management. 'There is evidence of a lessening dependence on physicians in some parts of the world and a related strengthening of various paramedical and auxiliary groups' (WHO Sixth Report 1980:3).

(xvii) The imbalance in the provision of health care facilities. There is widespread agreement that:

> a better balance is needed between facilities at various levels, typically consisting of the subcentre (or clinic/dispensary), the health centre, and the district or rural hospital . . . The limited coverage offered by hospitals in any event makes it absolutely essential that a strong brake should be placed on the further development of large hospitals so as to permit the rapid expansion of a network of primary care institutions (WHO Sixth Report I 1980:3).

(xviii) Lack of appreciation of the fact that:

> the availability of extensive funds for health care does not itself ensure the existence of a system of care that will be accessible to all in keeping

with priority needs, as seen by both the health workers who provide the care and those who receive it . . . There is a growing consensus that additional expenditure on health care, at least in the developed countries, is not bringing about a commensurate improvement in health (WHO Sixth Report I 1980:3).

It is now widely agreed that a pattern of spending heavily biased towards technically sophisticated in-patient care is inappropriate, even in wealthy countries with their own particular disease problems. The issue is still more clear-cut in the case of low income countries:

Studies of the financing of health care systems are being extended by examination of the relationships between particular forms of financing and the provision of care in keeping with the priority need for primary health care coverage of the whole population (WHO Sixth Report I 1980:3).

(xix) Lack of appreciation of the fact that the thrust to achieve health care for all must be directed towards primary health care within the broader concept of family health. The family health system includes maternal and child care, care of the adolescent, care of the worker and care of the aged, with ramifications into the more specialised aspects of this work according to individual needs and situations. The main support system of an effective primary health care system is the community, its family units and its social systems. Health workers tend to overlook the role of the family in the provision of health care. This is a disastrous mistake. The family is the nucleus of the community. Family-focused health care lies at the heart of community involvement.

Specific background issues

Poverty

WHO health experts agree that the last decade has been a difficult one for the improvement of world health. Droughts and severe winters have reduced livestock and harvests. Wars and civil unrest have destroyed crops, land, housing and the economy. The problem of refugees from a number of countries is a major one.

Increased inflation has added to the poverty of millions of people. It is estimated that 300 million breadwinners in the world are unemployed. At least 800 million people in the developing world live in a state of profound deprivation of the basic necessities for sustaining life. Their incomes barely support life and they have little (and frequently no) access to health services. At least 450 million people do not have the food to maintain basic survival. Life is shortened by an insidious starvation process. Less than a third of the people in all the underdeveloped countries have safe water and sanitation facilities. Housing conditions are deplorable. The urban drift is preventing many from erecting homes according to traditional methods, for example mud and reed structures. Tin and cardboard shanties provide shelter. The results are slums, social disorder and disease.

It is clear that educational facilities in the underdeveloped countries cannot keep pace with their abnormal population growth, resulting in an ever-growing illiteracy rate among adults.

Population size and growth

According to WHO, the annual rate of the population increase between 1970 and 1977 was 2,7% in Latin America, 2,7% in Africa, 2,6% in South Asia, and 1% in North America and Europe. The world population now increases by approximately 80 million persons annually. Ten years ago this figure was approximately 68 million.

The birth rate in the underdeveloped countries of the world ranges between 26 and 49 per 1 000, while in the developed countries it varies from 15 to 19 per 1 000. The death rate varies from 9 to 23 per 1 000 in the less developed countries and from 7 to 11 per 1 000 in the developed countries. This imbalance between the birth and death rates results in population growth. In the underdeveloped regions of the world this is a serious matter, for population growth exercises tremendous pressure on a nation's economy.

> A large number of infants and young children have to be fed and cared for. Later they will need to be educated or trained, and later still jobs will be needed for them as they enter the labour force. The provision of public and individual health services is only one of many competing demands. Rapid population increase often results in increases in the number of people living in poverty, the number uneducated, the number underfed. People in these categories are usually in poorer health and have greater need of health services . . . the need for health services increases at the same time as the ability to meet that need is strained (WHO Sixth Report I 1980:11).

Curbing population growth is the basis of social and economic development in the third world. The remedy for their poverty and social inequality lies in the hands of the people of these countries. The belief that other countries which have controlled their population growth owe them financial assistance is a false ideology.

In less developed communities mortality rates for women are higher in the reproductive ages than they are for men at a comparable age level. This is mainly due to factors conducive to maternal mortality.

In 1975 more than a third of the world's population was below the age of 15 years. In the *less developed* countries the proportion of this group was 40% compared with 25% in the *more developed* countries, where the proportion of young people has declined, with a concomitant growth in the number of persons over the age of 65 years. According to WHO the child dependency ratio was almost 100% higher and the old-age dependency ratio nearly 60% lower in the less developed countries than in the developed countries (WHO Sixth Report I 1980:9-14).

Urban growth

One of the alarming features of population distribution throughout the world is the excessively rapid urbanisation rate. Between 1950 and 1975 the world's urban population more than doubled. At present it constitutes a staggering 39% of the total world population. In the less developed countries with more land space the urban population represents about 27% of the total population, whereas in the more developed countries with their high density populations the proportion is approximately 70%. Taken at face value this should not present any problems, but the process of urbanisation is far faster in the underdeveloped poor countries in the last 25 years has increased 300% where it has only increased 70% in the developed countries (WHO Sixth Report I 1980:14).

Migrant workers

There is considerable migration of workers between developed and developing countries.

> The ILO estimated in 1973 that there were about 11 million migrant workers in Europe, with an annual flow of 600 000 to 1 000 000, and about 4,2 million resident foreigners in Northern America. In Latin America, Argentina has perhaps 500 000 to 1 000 000 migrants from other countries and Venezuela 300 000 to 7 000 000. In Africa, Ghana and the Ivory Coast are estimated to have 900 000 to 1 000 000 migrants and South Africa and Southern Rhodesia (Zimbabwe) about 300 000 (WHO Sixth Report I 1980:15).

Refugees

It is estimated that there are about 4 000 000 refugees and displaced persons in Asia, 3 000 000 in Africa, 112 000 in Latin America, 152 000 in North America, 570 000 in Europe and 2 000 in Australia and New Zealand. Unstable political situations in many parts of the world are adding a steady stream of refugees to the foregoing figures (WHO Sixth Report I 1980:15).

The family unit

The family is the basic social unit for the renewal of mankind. It is within the family environment that children grow up and develop physically, psychologically and socially. The family also has responsibilities towards its sick, dependent and aged members. The family or the household is the primary unit in respect of housing needs, the consumption of durable goods, cost of living, savings, etc. It is also the most relevant unit upon which to base planning and marketing for future needs (WHO Sixth Report I 1980:16).

The family as the basic social cell has numerous implications for the planning and delivery of health care and for the utilisation of facilities. WHO attaches great importance to the family in relation to national health policies and strategies.

Food and nutrition

'While malnutrition is caused by an interplay of a large number of factors, the three main ones are food production and availability, economic situation and population which are closely interrelated' (WHO Sixth Report I 1980:18). Malnutrition occurs in two extremes: malnutrition due to affluence – overeating, etc, and malnutrition due to extreme poverty – hunger. Of the approximately 1 200 million people in Asia and Africa, at least one third to a half suffer from malnutrition. This is particularly so among the children in these countries. The problem in Latin America appears to be equally severe, although reliable statistics are not available.

Education

By 1977 approximately 80% of the adult population of developing countries were still illiterate. This represented 800 million people or one fifth of the world's population. No less than 60% of the world's adult illiterates are women! This has enormous implications for health education:

> The enormous increase in the number of children in the developing world has outpaced the increase in enrolment so that the absolute number of children who are not at school has continued to increase. Thus the number of illiterate adults will continue to increase as well (WHO Sixth Report I 1980:22).

Other factors

Apart from such factors as social change and economic factors, personal factors also have an impact on the health status of the world. Factors such as smoking, stress, ecological impact on health, cultural beliefs and practices, anxiety, alcoholism, drug abuse and sexual permissiveness make a major contribution to the morbidity and mortality profiles of the human race.

Health development is human development

Health has come to be regarded as an essential aspect of human development. A number of international organisations of the United Nations are concerned with health development issues. WHO and UNICEF, in particular, show a major interest in the development of sound health policies, focusing on the role of primary health care in the implementation of such policies. The World Bank, which provides funds for economic development programmes, also plays a part. The programme recommended by the United Nations Water Conference for the provision of safe water supplies and sanitation for all by the year 1990 could have a major impact on the promotion of health if it were to be implemented. However, it appears exceedingly doubtful that this will be possible.

The policy of UNEP for the protection of the environment and the UNESCO programme for raising literacy levels worldwide must inevitably benefit health development.

Health development is not an issue for health personnel alone. 'Health development both contributes to and results from social and economic development, hence health policies have to form a part of overall development policies' (WHO Sixth Report I 1980:52). WHO has elaborated two important fundamental principles for health development:

> One is that governments have responsibility for the health of their people, and that at the same time people should have the right, as well as the duty, individually and collectively, to participate in development of their own health.

> Governments and the health professions also have the duty of providing the public with the information and social framework that will enable them to assume greater responsibility for their own health . . . Self-reliance implies taking initiatives, determining what can be done without external resources when appropriate, and deciding when to seek external support for what purposes and from what sources . . . An important part of recent health policy has been the realization of the interdependence of individuals, communities and countries based on their common concern for health . . . The concept of social and economic productivity is based on the understanding that human

energy is the most important motive force for development and that health is the key to generating human energy required for development. The road to health and the road to development are the same.

Primary Health Care is regarded as the key to attaining the target of health for all by the year 2000 as a part of overall development and in the spirit of social justice (WHO Sixth Report I 1980:52-53).

Issues requiring attention

Issues requiring constant, more aggressive attention are the development of the data and information systems necessary for health planning, analysis of the current health care needs and situation, appropriate health legislation, the planning and implementation of suitable health care delivery systems, sound administrative practices, financing, health promotion and disease prevention and control (for example parasitic diseases, enteric infections, tuberculosis, leprosy, cerebrospinal meningitis, smallpox, diseases of childhood preventable by immunisation, viral diseases, zoonoses and foodborne diseases, sexually transmitted diseases, endemic treponematoses, blindness, cardiovascular diseases, cancer, respiratory diseases, diseases of genetic origin, diabetes mellitus, chronic rheumatic diseases and diseases of the structures of the oral cavity).

All countries should have sound policies for the control of environmental health with particular reference to the factors which influence or are influenced by the environment. Priorities in such a programme are maintaining the ecological balance of the soil biosystems and their environment, the conservation of water and control of the community water supply and of waste disposal, human settlements and housing, control of physical and chemical hazards in the environment and food safety.

In the field of family health more determined action is necessary regarding the promotion of maternal and child health, the reduction of maternal mortality and morbidity, infant and childhood morbidity and mortality, health care in adolescence, the utilisation of resources, manpower management and training, family planning, day care for children, school health, social legislation, nutritional development, health education, the health of the working population, the promotion of mental health, alcohol-related problems, drug dependence problems, psychosocial factors, mental health care, pharmaceutical control policies and supply, accident prevention and control and disasters and natural catastrophies. All these issues require unceasing vigilance in the form of a pragmatic approach by the policy makers and providers of health care, community involvement, dedication on the part of health workers and a willingness to form part of a broad team of community workers for the development of health care.

Health problem areas

WHO has identified a number of basic problems which obstruct the delivery of health care.

Financial resources

In the developed countries there have been major escalations in the cost of health care, yet the amount spent on health care in these countries is insignificant in relation to the amount spent on defence and education. The amount spent on health development remains fairly constant at between 5-6% of gross national expenditure.

In underdeveloped countries health expenditure amounts to 2-3% of gross national expenditure. Bearing in mind how low national expenditure generally is, this does not represent a generous allocation.

An important factor in the application of this expenditure is the fact that the health care industry is labour-intensive. Health manpower consumes between 60% to 80% of the health budget in most countries, with the result that very little 'is left over to provide the infrastructure and the non-labour inputs needed for health manpower to achieve optimum productivity' (WHO Sixth Report I 1980:180).

Faced with the ever-spiralling costs of health manpower, health planners are taking a serious look at the type of health personnel they now use:

> Within the constraints of a limited budget, it might be possible to decrease the proportion spent on health manpower by decreasing the emphasis on those health workers who are costly to train and maintain, and increasing the emphasis on the less costly categories (WHO Sixth Report I 1980:180).

Let this be a word of warning to registered nurses and midwives who are not delivering quality care. They will be replaced by semi-trained persons!

Lack of appropriate planning

There appears to be a worldwide lack of effective health planning as a continuous process, as well as of well-organised information systems. This leads to innumerable problems in health programme development, for example maldistribution of available health resources, increased reliance on expensive health care technology, scant coverage of health needs, ineffective logistics and a host of other problems. One of the main problems concerns health manpower needs. Inadequate planning leads to:

> shortages of appropriately trained teachers and supervisors, appropriate teaching and learning materials, and facilities for training; inappropriate curricula and standards for recruitment to training and employment; a lack of security of tenure and of career-development schemes, including a lack of the continuing education needed to increase work productivity and job satisfaction and to facilitate the vertical and horizontal mobility of health workers; a lack of schemes for the appropriate distribution of health workers geographically, institutionally, and by occupation; and a lack of clear definitions of the functions and tasks of health team members. All these deficiencies combine to create shortages of certain categories of health personnel having the knowledge, skills and attitudes needed to perform the work (WHO Sixth Report I 1980:181).

It is a simple statistical fact that there is a great imbalance in the distribution of basic health manpower in the world. It is estimated that in the developed countries there are about 1 000 health workers for every 100 000 inhabitants, while in the underdeveloped countries there are about 200 per 100 000. This is due not only to financial stringency, but also to the low level of social and economic development in many countries. It must also be noted that the potential health care contribution of the 200 health workers per 100 000 of population is reduced significantly by such factors as maldistribution of health personnel, low density of population distribution and poor communication systems. It is interesting to note that in the developed countries there are six times as many physicians, five times as many pharmacists and 12 times as many nurses and midwives per 100 000 as there are in the developing countries, and in many developing countries physician density is declining. This necessitates an acceleration in the production of middle and lower level health personnel. In addition to the problem of the scarcity of physicians is their maldistribution: they are largely urban-based health manpower. Tragically, this trend is current among Black nurses in South Africa.

Health manpower planning

Here is disillusionment with planning methods that calls for isolated, sophisticated, and costly studies in which more data are generally collected than can be meaningfully used and certain essential data are omitted either because data gathering is badly organized or because the national information system is incapable of generating the data needed. Such studies have seldom resulted in the formulation and implementation of a plan (WHO Sixth Report I 1980:185).

As a result crash planning research is being developed, using simplified techniques for gauging manpower requirements. The growing number of categories of health personnel and the number of grades of such personnel complicate the issue.

Currently there is great concern about the growing cost of health manpower education. Worldwide it is being asked whether the increases in the complexity and the cost of the education of health workers are commensurate with improvements in the level of health of the community. This is a vital issue which all professions must examine. Rising salaries will inevitably result in the utilisation of lower paid categories of worker.

Health manpower education

During the last three decades the traditional education of health workers has consistently been accused of failing to meet the needs of society and of emphasising the wrong priorities in its curricula. For some years now WHO has been advocating a system of education of health professionals that cuts across traditional approaches. Among these are:

the multi-disciplinary (health team) approach to education and training; the inclusion in curricula of aspects of the social and behavioural sciences as a foundation for participation in comprehensive community health as opposed to curative medicine for the individual; interspersion of theoretical with practical training; student oriented rather than teacher oriented instruction; learning on the job; learning by doing; self-instruction; problem oriented instruction; the modularization of curricula; the flow-chart system for enhancing skills and facilitating decision-making in patient management by intermediate-level health staff and peripheral health workers, such as traditional birth attendants and primary health care workers; packaged instruction; teaching and learning by task oriented behavioural objectives; individual and small-group learning systems; and the evaluation of student performance and of the whole teaching and learning process (WHO Sixth Report I 1980:188).

Task analysis as a guide to the specification of contemplated skill requirements and thus of learning objectives is the foundation for the planning of curricula for health manpower training. WHO personnel believe that 'the nursing profession has played a pioneering role in the development of methodology for the evaluation of education programmes in the health field' (WHO Sixth Report I 1980:189).

Health manpower management

The management of health manpower incorporates all matters relating to the recruitment, employment, use and motivation of all categories of health worker. It largely ensures the productivity and coverage of the health system. The major symptoms of poor health manpower management are the uneconomical use of staff, resulting in low productivity, imbalances in the composition of the labour force and maldistribution of health manpower within the health system in terms of geographical and functional aspects. Poor manpower planning is basic to poor manpower management. It is interesting to note that the statistics available to WHO indicate that in the developed countries there is an average of 100 doctors to 294 other health workers, whereas in the underdeveloped countries this ratio is 100 to 489. These are average figures for the developed regions and the underdeveloped regions. In many countries the ratio is even more unsatisfactory than the average for all underdeveloped regions.

Measures to ensure optimal productivity of health care personnel are essential, but are not generally applied due to the lack of health personnel trained in health management practice.

Problems regarding the provision of post-graduate and post-basic continuing education opportunities continue to plague the developing countries, where a shortage of teaching personnel with high level knowledge of local conditions, the speciality concerned and educational principles and strategies bedevils the issue.

Physician and nurse migration from the developing to the developed countries is a major problem for the countries of origin of these health workers. Poor countries spend a lot of money on educating and training health personnel, only to find that they lose the personnel to the developed countries. In 1972 there were 140 000 migrant doctors in the USA, Canada, the United Kingdom, the Federal Republic of Germany and Australia. A large number of these came from the developing countries, although a substantial number moved from countries in Europe. The loss of nursing personnel from the developing countries through migration cannot readily be estimated, although it is considered to be in excess of the figures pertaining to doctors. Many of the developed countries are now exercising more stringent immigration control to curb the movement of health personnel from the developing countries. The need to develop the educational opportunities for health personnel in their countries of origin is a constant one.

Health care facilities

Generally the health care facilities in the developing countries are of three basic types – the regional or district hospital, the health centre and the health station (clinic or dispensary or one-man subcentre). Hospitals are divided into national referral or consultant hospitals, regional hospitals, and district or rural hospitals. Theoretically the hospitals in a country should be linked in a network with each other, each hospital's capacity (number of beds and facilities) being related to its particular catchment area. This is seldom the case in the developing countries. Weaknesses in the primary health care system and in the capacity of the health centres (as well as in the ability of the workers at this level) still results in over-crowded hospitals.

The tendency to neglect the development of basic rural health services is very evident in the manner in which clinics are placed, staffed and sup-plied with essential medical and nursing supplies.

The tendency to erect massive buildings equipped with advanced tech-nological facilities persists, despite the fact that the maintenance of such facilities swallows the greater portion of the available health finances. In the erection of expensive hospitals little attention seems to be given to the lower level institutions and services which exist or are needed in the health care network.

The tendency to keep patients in hospital longer than is necessary per-sists because often it is not possible to discharge them as they have nowhere to go or because there is no subsidiary health support service to take on the further care that may be necessary. Many patients from country areas could be treated on an out-patients basis if hostel accom-modation was available to them. It is for this reason that decentralisation of health care facilities is so important, for such patients could be catered for in health centres, clinics and by community (including occupational health) nurses.

Hostel accommodation at hospitals is an essential feature of modern hospital planning in developing countries. It is well-established in many rural South African hospitals, as well as in the maternity centres in rural areas. It constitutes a saving not only in respect of the erection and main-tenance of hospital buildings, but also in respect of staff and supplies.

Distribution of beds

This remains a thorny issue. Bed occupancy rates vary widely from country to country. Much depends on the nature and quality of the health services available, the social and economic situation in the country, the distances patients have to travel to reach a health care facility, the cul-tural attitudes of the population and the number of health service per-sonnel available.

Financing health care

The most common financing mechanisms are personal payment, chari-table donations, free service to indigents, payment by employers, volun-tary insurance (medical aid schemes) and social insurance (national health schemes), tax appropriations and community self-help efforts. Through-out the world, in both developed and underdeveloped countries, the problem of financing health care is an acute one.

Research

'Health research is critically important for the achievement of national development goals, and developing countries need to build up a research potential' (WHO Sixth Report I 1980:206). A portion of the finances available for health care must always be made available for research. Organisation of research activities in the health field falls into four major categories, namely:

(i) research by a central body charged with the responsibility of defining objectives and assigning priorities, for example the Medical Research Council in South Africa (a variety of organisations, both government and non-government, are involved in the process)

(ii) international research cooperation

(iii) individual, privately financed research

(iv) research conducted at the local level by a health care institution and which does not form part of the national programmes financed and approved by the central body.

The latter two types of research are of great importance for improvements in the quality of the service at local level, for identifying specific health needs and constraints in the area, and for increasing the potential of the service as a whole as well as of particular categories of personnel. They present endless opportunities for studying health care delivery at the point of impact – the community. At all these levels of research organisation the disease factors, the diagnostic and therapeutic factors, the facilities, the health manpower factors, the health service management factors, the cost-efficiency factors, the socio-cultural-economic factors, the distribution factors and the preventive, promotive, curative and rehabilitative factors, as well as the logistics factors, can be studied.

The Declaration of Alma Ata, adopted on 12 September 1978 by the International Conference on Primary Health Care which was jointly sponsored by WHO and UNICEF, clearly states that primary health care is the key to attaining the goal of health for all by the year 2000. The Declaration calls on all governments to formulate national policies, strategies and plans of action for the provision of primary health care as part of a comprehensive national health system in coordination with other sectors. The Declaration also calls for international action to achieve this goal.

What is meant by health for all? The concept will be interpreted differently by different countries in the light of their social and economic characteristics, health status, the morbidity patterns of its population and state of development of its health system. A general understanding of the concept implies that every individual should have access to primary health care and through this to all levels of a comprehensive health system. Fundamental to this is the objective of continuous improvement of the health of individuals and the community as a whole. Social and economic development is an essential component of the strategy to achieve the goal. The achievement of the goal through the provision of primary health care requires *at least* the following:

> Education concerning prevailing health problems and the methods of preventing and controlling them; promotion of food supply and proper nutrition; an adequate supply of safe water and basic sanitation, maternal and child care, including family planning; immunization against the major infectious diseases; prevention and control of locally endemic diseases; appropriate treatment of common diseases and injuries and provision of essential drugs (WHO 1979:12).

WHO envisages:

> that the planning, organization and operation of primary health care is a long-term process and total population coverage by it may have to be achieved in stages. An essential feature is that is should be extended progressively in both geographical coverage and content until it covers the entire population with all essential components (1979:13).

Implementation of action to attain the goals

According to WHO, each country requires at least the following in order to attain the goal of health for all by the year 2000:

(i) A national health policy determined in accordance with its overall socio-economic development policy and taking into consideration its own problems, possibilities, circumstances, social and economic structures, and political and administrative systems.

(ii) National strategies which include the systematic identification and use of suitable entry points for developing health potential and the involvement of other sectors concerned with socio-economic, managerial and technical development. The identification of favourable factors as well as possible obstacles and constraints and the development of strategies to deal with these are essential.

(iii) Political commitment through political decisions which enable socio-economic development and health care development to proceed hand-in-hand.

(iv) Social policies which aim at improving the quality of life and maximum health benefits for all.

(v) Community participation so that communities can assume greater responsibility for their own health and welfare, including self-care. This is a social, economic and technical necessity. Much community education will be needed to achieve this input.

(vi) Administrative reform, with the emphasis on strengthening and adapting administrative structures and systems at all levels and in all sectors with well-planned inter-sectoral coordination between health and education, agriculture, food production, water resource control, housing and environmental protection. Delegation of authority for some of these levels of activity is essential.

(vii) Finances, with the emphasis on the reallocation of resources so that health care obtains a fair share of the national budget. Emphasis on the utilisation of local resources and supplies as far as possible to meet health requirements is essential, since this is financially advantageous.

(viii) Enabling legislation to allow action to be taken at the various government and non-government levels by the community and health personnel.

(ix) National plans of action with clear objectives and clear guidelines regarding *what* has to be done, *who* has to do it, *when* it has to be done, *where* it has to be done and *how* it has to be done. This will involve health care system design, programme development, process development, information systems development, evaluation process design, training in health management and the establishment of national health councils and national centres for health development.

It would also include such aspects as the identification of the basis for health development action in a region, the nature of the essential health programmes and services, the type of community support and coverage necessary, the appropriate technology, health manpower development and training, the development of referral systems, the development of facilities and logistic support and control, health research, reorientation of the existing health system, identification and development of the type of support that can be provided from other sectors, the development of guidelines and the monitoring and evaluation of the programmes.

Implementation of a global strategy

Cooperation by countries at a regional level must be encouraged so that cooperation at an international level for the implementation of a global strategy by WHO becomes possible. This global strategy is concerned with:

   (i) the promotion at the highest government and non-government levels of 'the idea that an acceptable level of health for all by the year 2000 is feasible' (WHO 1979:41)
  (ii) the strengthening of global mechanisms for attracting bilateral and multilateral funds and for ensuring that they are channelled into priority activities in countries (*ibid*:41)
 (iii) the provision of a global information exchange system
  (iv) the provision of a global system of technical cooperation among developing countries
   (v) the provision of global orientation and support for research
  (vi) the fostering of global use of expertise available in the member countries
 (vii) the development of a system of global monitoring and evaluation
(viii) the utilisation of a more effective role for WHO in promotion, coordination, supplying information, technical cooperation and monitoring and evaluation
  (ix) the preparation of a time framework in terms of which planned action should be carried out.

Development of indicators for monitoring progress

An important task of national planners is to develop *health indicators* for the measurement of progress towards health for all by the year 2000.

WHO envisages that there should be *four categories of indicators*:
 (i) health policy indicators
 (ii) social and economic indicators
(iii) indicators of the provision of health care
(iv) indicators of health status, including the quality of life.

Interpretation of the goal

In May 1977 the Thirtieth World Health Assembly adopted resolution WHA 30, 43 in which it was decided that:

the main social target of governments and of WHO in the coming decades should be the attainment by all the people of the world by the year 2000 of a level of health that will permit them to lead a socially and economically productive life. This is popularly known as 'health for all by the year 2000' (WHO 1981a:15).

Dr H Mahler, Director-General of WHO, made it clear that the concept 'Health for all by the year 2000' does not mean that:

there will be no sick or disabled by the year 2000, nor does it mean that there will be doctors and nurses to provide health care for all by the year 2000 . . . it does mean that people will realize that they themselves have the power to shape their lives and the lives of their families, free from the avoidable burden of disease, aware that ill-health is not inevitable. It does mean that people will use better approaches than they do now for preventing disease and alleviating unavoidable illness and disability, and better ways of growing up and growing old, and dying gracefully. It does mean that there will be an even distribution among the population of whatever health resources are available. And it does mean that essential health care will be accessible to all individuals and families, in an acceptable and affordable way, and with their full involvement (WHO 1981b:79).

Bringing the potential of health by the year 2000 to all is one of the great ideals of mankind. It is recognised that it will be difficult to attain, but what is difficult is not necessarily impossible. A concerted effort by the governments and peoples of the world could make this a realisable proposition. WHO believes that it is realisable through the adoption of the concept of specific global targets within the broad concept of primary health care. These global targets are important. They relate specifically to the essential *minimal list* of the primary health care concept. These global targets are the following:

(i) Everyone in every country will have ready access to essential health care and to first level referral facilities.

(ii) Everyone will be actively involved in caring for themselves and their families as far as they can and in community action for health.

(iii) Communities throughout the world will share with their governments responsibility for the health care of their members.

(iv) All governments will have assumed overall responsibility for the health of their people.

(v) Safe drinking water and sanitation will be available to all people.

(vi) All people will be adequately nourished.

(vii) All children will be immunised against the major infectious diseases of childhood.

(viii) Communicable diseases in the developing countries will be of no greater public health significance in the year 2000 than they are in developed countries in the year 1980.

(ix) All possible means will be applied to prevent and control communicable diseases and promote mental health through influencing lifestyle and controlling the physical and psychosocial environment.

(x) Essential drugs will be available to all.

The role of nurses (including midwives)

The nurse in the primary health care field has four roles to fulfil, namely that of provider of primary health care in clinics, in homes and in industry;

supervisor of nurses and other primary health care workers; teacher of nurses and other primary health care workers; and manager of nursing services, which include a network of primary health care facilities.

It is essential that the nurse in a leadership role understands the health care needs and constraints of the area or region she serves, as well as the national health care situation. Nurses in top level nursing management and nursing education positions must have a broad knowledge of the health care situation in surrounding countries, as well as some knowledge of the international health care scene.

The world pandemic of Aids will make the ideal of health for all by the year 2000 unattainable.

References and general bibliography

FAO Production Yearbook Vol. 31. 1978. Rome FAO.

Fülop, T. 1978. New approaches to a permanent problem – the integrated development of health services and health manpower. *WHO Chronicle*, 30: 433-471.

Hall, TL & Mejia, A. (Eds). 1978. *Health manpower planning: principles, methods and issues*. Geneva: WHO.

Hornby, P, Ray, DK, Shipp, PJ & Hall, TL. 1980. *Guidelines for health manpower planning*. Geneva: WHO.

ILO. 1973. *Migrant Labourers*. International Labour Conference Report VII (I). Geneva: ILO.

UNO. 1978. *Report of the United Nations Commissioner for Refugees to the General Assembly, 33rd Session*. New York: UNO.

WHO. 1971. *The development of studies in health manpower*. Technical Report Series No 481. Geneva: WHO.

WHO. 1978. *Bulletin of the WHO*, 56.

WHO. 1978. *Financing of health services*. Technical Report Series No 625. Geneva: WHO.

WHO. 1979. *Formulating strategies for health for all by the year 2000*. Geneva: WHO.

WHO. 1980. *Sixth Report on the World Health Situation Part I*. Geneva: WHO.

WHO. 1980. *Sixth Report on the World Health Situation Part II*. Geneva: WHO.

WHO. 1981a. *Global strategy for health for all by the year 2000*. Geneva: WHO.

WHO. 1981b. *WHO Chronicle*, Geneva: WHO.

WHO. 1981c. *World Health Statistics Annual*. Geneva: WHO.

World Health Organisation and United Nations Childrens Fund. 1978. *Alma Ata. Primary Health Care*. Geneva: WHO.

PART 6

Some aspects of nursing education

12

The academic in the nursing profession

Introductory commentary

Many professional women have asked: what is the role of the academic in the nursing profession? Nurse tutor courses have been available in South African universities for more than 50 years (since 1937), while degree courses for nurses have been available since 1956. Nurse educationists have planned these courses, been responsible for their acceptance at university level and been involved in their teaching since 1937, yet doctors, professional women from other professions and educational policy-makers still ask: what is the role of the academic in the nursing profession? The role of the nurse academic in the development of the modern ethos of nursing is such a vital one that nurses find it difficult to understand why this question is asked. It is possibly as a result of the commonly held view that all nursing activities take place at the bedside and that nurses do not need formal education, but only experiential learning. It probably arises from a total misconception of what nursing is.

The question has been asked so frequently and in so many countries that the matter was presented at an International Symposium for Women held at Grahamstown in the seventies.

THE ADDRESS

Introduction

In their efforts to provide higher education for nurses, nurse academics have made a contribution to the cause of women within the higher education system in South Africa. Too few women in this country have reached professional status. In some of the universities which have established a department of nursing nurse academics were the first women to be appointed to a Chair and the first women to secure a seat on the senate of a university. These lone figures, through their good sense and sound academic ability, have won the unstinting support of their fellow academics.

In some universities there was discrimination against the permanent appointment and the academic advancement of married women. Nurse academics waged a relentless war against this discrimination and finally won the fight, not only for nurses, but for married women in all academic disciplines.

Seeing that the nurse academic is a recent addition to the health team in South Africa, and that currently all the nurse academics in this country are women, it is an appropriate time to look at some aspects of their role.

Like her counterpart and colleague, the academic in the medical profession, the nurse academic is a searcher for and a transmitter of knowledge, an identifier and an interpreter of what has been, what is, and what is likely to be in a particular professional discipline or section of that discipline. She is a knowledge worker. Nurse academics have to identify and interpret the nature of nursing in all its diverse dimensions, the influence of its heritage on the present and on the future, and how all this is affected by the society in which it exists. The role of the nurse academic must be seen against the background of the contribution of the great historical figures in nursing, who were not only remarkable nurses, but women of great stature in their respective nations. History has accorded many of them honoured places in its halls of fame.

Professional nursing was born under the triple influence of religion, military needs and science. From these sources it has inherited three great concepts – *charity, discipline* and *learning*. Through time the great women who have left a lasting imprint on nursing succeeded in passing on these priceless concepts, which have become the cornerstone of the professional nursing edifice, to their successors. In this year of the woman nurses must pay tribute to the long line of distinguished women who not only served nursing with great success, but made a great impact on the social engineering systems of their respective nations.

These were the women who worked towards the ideal of taking nursing education into the universities and who gave the academics in nursing the injunction that central to their teaching should be the age-old concepts of *charity, discipline* and *learning*, interpreted in their contemporary context. It is their recognition of the fact that the spirit of learning will conquer (*vincet anima doctrinae*) that has brought academics into the nursing profession in so many parts of the world.

The task of the academic

The view presented here of what constitutes the task of the academic in nursing is coloured by the views of the leaders of nursing in South Africa, who for a century have struggled to provide this country with a competent nursing service. In the process they strove to provide opportunities for university education for nurses in their own country. The profession pays special tribute to this group for their vision, their determination, their teaching, their ability to identify priorities and their ability to identify what has meaning for nursing, not only in the present, but also in the future.

The nurse academic stands not only at the crossroads of time, but also at the convergence of conflicting views and different outlooks on the professional roles of the present, the past, and the future, which make the task of teaching and healing complicated and contentious. As interpreter of a discipline which so closely affects man's welfare she has to explore, examine, test and evaluate these divergent viewpoints and interpret them to a profession in which change is so rapid in some respects that its today is already its yesterday. This is a difficult and challenging task. However, challenge is part of the everyday life of the nurse, so the nurse academic will accept this new challenge.

Charity

Her concept of charity in nursing, that is the element of concern and love for mankind, will play a decisive role in how the nurse academic tackles the tasks ahead. It will be decisive in how she plumbs her own resources to meet the challenges of today as if it is already tomorrow. To achieve this she needs the drive to extend her own knowledge and the mental and physical resilience to withstand the pace. Fundamental to her success as a teacher is her own philosophy about the discipline she interprets and her own goals in life. Fundamental, too, is her philosophy about our responsibility as human beings to be concerned for our fellow men. This is important!

The practice of the healing arts is the oldest specialised activity characteristic of all cultures. Because all of mankind is concerned about health, international cooperation in health matters has always been fruitful. The World Health Organisation (WHO) maintains that the health of all peoples is fundamental to the attainment of peace and security. Health professionals are becoming acutely aware that efforts to improve the health of a people have a positive effect on the socio-economic development of the community. In a world in which there is still a great deal of poverty, at both the domestic and the international levels, health services are increasingly being incorporated in the social engineering services aimed at improving man's total welfare. The nurse academic has to prepare her students for this. Of great importance is the international cooperation which comes so readily to health professionals.

The concept charity has always been interpreted in nursing as concern and love for one's fellow men. This is vital in international health work. Hence health professionals, of whom nurses constitute the greatest number, may ultimately, through their international efforts for man's health and their charity concern and love, achieve the universally desired goal of world health and, indirectly, world peace.

The nurse academic's philosophy, her interpretation of the concept charity, her research and its interpretation, should all be aimed at achieving this universal goal. Health care builds bridges between nations, cultures and individuals. Women are in the forefront of this thrust. This gives a new dimension to the concept 'charity'.

With concern and love for their fellow men as the basis, the nurse academic's task is to motivate and guide her students to develop into the type of professionals the international health scene needs. Through her writings and research and participation in the affairs of the nation she has to make her profession, and the society of which she forms part, aware of the end goals for human development through health. In all this she must highlight the possibilities for international understanding and cooperation through cooperation in health matters.

She must also discover and help develop leaders, researchers and writers for the nursing profession. More important than this is her fundamental task of helping her students to establish a philosophical baseline of their own. She has to help them to explore and evaluate the knowledge they will require to cope with the demands of the present and the future. As co-explorer and interpreter the nurse academic must help identify and interpret all that is relevant to the practice of contemporary nursing. She has to see this relevance in a situation in which new knowledge about the natural and biological sciences, technological development, social change, political uncertainty and the upheaval of old established values are all having a profound influence on the provision of health care. She has to expound this relevance where excessive pursuit of material gains and adherence to material values leave little time for the humanistic values, and where the 'give me, give me' attitudes of a seeking society tend to erode man's emotional and physical health, despite the provision of extensive health care.

An important task of the nurse academic is to support the student or professional colleague who is torn between conforming with the new type of social collectivism which is stripped of the responsibility to exercise freedom with responsibility and conforming with her own professional philosophical outlook which sees meaning in man's life and hence in individual responsibility. This is no easy matter. Somehow the nurse academic has to find the courage and the will to help those who are thinking their way through their own dilemmas and to recognise that individual man has responsibility for his own acts and omissions and for the quality of his own life, for this is the basis of health, of all planning in health, and of charity in whatever guise it presents.

Her most important task is to help lay a foundation of personal and professional philosophy which will enable her students, and those other members of her profession whose lives she influences, to live in society as individuals, as professionals, as stable members of the community and as nation builders. To achieve this ideal, the work of the nurse academic is directed at helping her young colleagues, in both the teaching/learning situation and the broader sphere of professional practice, to develop the ability and the will to work in a team, to assume responsibilities, and to do this with critical thinking, self-respect, and respect for the dignity, rights and freedom of others. At the same time she has to help them to a belief in the worthwhileness of the job. In a role which has international implications, she has the task to help them to develop confidence with humility, resourcefulness, the ability to adjust to new situations, leadership potential, the ability to reason and the ability to debate a point of view, either verbally or in writing.

Because youth is impatient for action, one of the tasks of the nurse academic is to lead her young colleague in the modern university setting to the realisation that inculcated knowledge is not enough; she also needs personal life experience. She must evaluate and synthesise these aspects if she is to develop into a sound practitioner and citizen. The development of the student's creative abilities and personality and of her understanding of her role in the community and society at large is of great importance.

If the nurse academic interprets the ethos of nursing and its present and future roles with sensitivity, she should be able to cultivate in her students a love of the cultural heritage of the profession and its aesthetic and moral values. If she herself has a yearning for the fundamental truths which underlie her profession, for justice, honesty, self-respect and respect for others, and for the ability and the opportunity to serve, in their search for role identification her students will reach out to these values.

If she can convey to them that moral and spiritual values will enable them to live with dignity in contemporary society, in which changing values and knowledge and technological explosions have become major forces which shape the lives of men, she will have done well. If she is able to inculcate in them a sensitivity to basic human and professional values, and if she can lead them to see meaning in living as individual human being rather than unidentifiable parts of a mass society, she is doing better still. She will have done society proud if she can help them to understand how to use their rational powers to recall, generalise, compare, imagine, classify, analyse, synthesise, deduce and infer, so that they can base their choices and their actions on understandings which they themselves have achieved and on values which they themselves have analysed. They will then see for themselves the consequences to others, and to themselves, of their use of their knowledge, their service and their value judgements. If she can help them to perceive and understand the events of their own lives and time, and the forces which influence these events, if she can help them to re-examine the status of man whom they serve, and if she can lead them to an understanding of the eroding effects of man's inability to cope with the everyday pressures of today's world, she will have put them on the path of true professionalism and citizenship.

Educated, useful citizens are part of the true capital resources of a nation. The nurse academic is making her contribution to the national treasury of human resources.

Discipline

Because charity spells concern and love, it requires disciples who are prepared to discipline themselves so that they may serve mankind. Discipline is something which is caught, not taught.

Recognition by the nursing professional that a disciplined mind is essential to cope with the demands of a profession the ramifications of which are as diverse as man's mental and physical needs, constitutes a basic requirement for both learning and practice. It is the particular task of the nurse academic, living in a society which bucks discipline, to convey to students, professional colleagues and John Citizen that disciplined forces are necessary in the fight for life and for man's total well-being. Self-discipline of a high order is necessary to acquire the knowledge that will enable the professional nurse to analyse and evaluate the value system of her profession and of her community, to see their implications for man's welfare, to see the need for health care, and to provide the service *when*, *where* and *how* it is needed. Self-discipline is essential for carrying on under emotionally traumatic conditions or in situations which threaten one's life. Self-discipline is necessary to enable one to care for one's enemy as if he were one's brother, or to see need and to provide service to those in need, irrespective of their social, political, economic, ethnic, cultural or religious status, of their colour, or of the sickness from which they suffer. The nurse academic prepares the seedbed for such disciplined behaviour, nurtures it and reinforces it by precept and example and by her writings. Acceptance by the student body is facilitated if the profession as a whole prescribes discipline as one of the criteria for quality nursing and for citizenship.

Learning

The third concept which nurse leaders have handed down to this generation of nurses is the concept that learning for professional service is something which extends over the entire working life of the practitioner. The nurse academic has to provide guidance in this respect through her research, her organisation of facilities, and her teaching contribution.

In this context I do not wish to deal with the content of courses. It must be emphasised that nurse academics have grave responsibility to ensure that all course content is relevant to the needs of the day. Furthermore, it is their duty to ensure that it is geared to providing a base for the entire working life of the professional nurse. Without this there can be no insight into future service needs, nor can post-graduate and continuing education programmes achieve their objectives.

Post-graduate education is as necessary in nursing as in any other discipline. The calibre of such education will have a profound influence on nursing and on the health services. Similarly, continuing education is a fundamental need of all nurses in practice. With regard to post-graduate and continuing education programmes, nurse academics have five areas of responsibility, namely:

(i) to bring about changes in negative attitudes

(ii) to introduce new concepts

(iii) to update knowledge and introduce new fields of knowledge

(iv) to serve society by assisting with the self-education of nurses

(v) to establish a scientific basis and a conceptual framework for the varied aspects of these learning situations.

It is the nurse academic who through research will identify the important parameters of post-graduate and continuing education. For this she should be an innovator and an identifier of the criteria which will determine the range and effectiveness of the programmes. She will have to assess the measure of accountability of both academic and learner in this process. It is recognition of this accountability which has influenced nurse academics in South Africa to work with other nurse leaders to identify:

(i) the need for further education of nurses

(ii) the need of the community for persons with such education

(iii) the problems of the nurse who is unable to attend a residential university

(iv) the ways in which these needs could be met.

The recent establishment of a department of nursing science in a teletuition university, the University of South Africa (UNISA), bears testimony to the drive and hopes of nurse academics and other nurse leaders in South Africa. These women have had the vision to tackle a professional and a community need by introducing an additional educational system for nursing which may at this stage be regarded as decidedly innovative in character. Their belief in the ability of the registered nurse to benefit from self-study under guidance, and that something should be done about meeting the needs of persons who as a result of their social commitments are not able to attend residential universities, lies behind the introduction of the external nursing degree courses at UNISA. Their vision and faith will benefit the nurses of Africa and the communities in which they live.

Enrolments already indicate that this benefit will extend to nurses in other parts of the world. The philosophy underlying nursing taught at residential universities is now being carried to the remote corners of our country and elsewhere, where nurses are recognising the need to be better equipped so that they may serve better. With rapid expansion of the role of the nurse in Africa this is grassroots social engineering. The output of students from this degree course justifies the experiment.

The emphasis has fallen on the identifying and interpreting role of the academic. She cannot fulfil this unless she does research to complement her knowledge and to help others to augment their knowledge. Research is the foundation of her academic endeavour and of her service to her profession and the community. It is the means which enables her to prepare her students and her profession to work within a health team at the inter-professional, inter-disciplinary and inter-occupational levels. Through her research and participation in health and social engineering she helps to serve in a comprehensive national and international health programme, to provide a service which cares for the health of mankind in all its dimensions at the preventive, promotive, curative and rehabilitative levels so that he may at some time experience the dream of total health, that is mental, physical and social well-being and not merely the absence of disease. When the attainment by all peoples of the highest levels of health, irrespective of race, religion, political beliefs and economic or social conditions is achieved, women, who constitute approximately 99% of the nursing force in the world, will have their reward for their years of devotion to a cause of this magnitude, and the nurse academic will have earned the tribute 'well-done thou good and faithful servant of mankind'.

13

Higher education for nurses by means of degrees or diplomas obtained through extramural, external or teletuition studies

Introductory commentary

When reading nursing literature some nurses become confused about the meaning of extramural, external and teletuition studies. Some clarification of these concepts is necessary and the impact of teletuition study on the development of the nursing profession in South Africa needs to be explored. This address attempts to examine the issue. A further overview will have to be done in 1990 and in 2000 AD.

THE ADDRESS

Introduction

Many countries are extending their higher education facilities for nurses by means of extramural (off-campus) degree and diploma courses, or by means of external degrees.

Some countries have instituted national statutory bodies to award degrees or diplomas to students who have followed approved courses of study at educational institutions other than universities, or who have studied entirely on their own. An example of a statutory body which awards degrees and which is not a university is the Council for National Academic Awards (CNAA) of Great Britain. A similar body exists in Australia for granting degrees to persons who complete applied science degree courses at colleges for Advanced Education. Nursing councils are statutory bodies authorised to award certificates and diplomas, that is they offer national awards.

External and extramural degrees

Let us differentiate briefly between extramural or off-campus degree courses and external degrees. The degrees are the same as those offered at residential universities. Where learning takes place gives the course its title. True extramural courses are those offered on a campus which is maintained by a parent university, but does not form part of the main campus. It may be located at a great distance from the parent university. The students may or may not be admitted to the rights and privileges of the student body on the main campus. Personnel appointed by the university undertake the teaching, or personnel from the parent university

111

teach at the extramural campus as required. The essence of the system is that the parent university provides a well-developed teaching programme and the students earn credits for the work of the academic year. There is face-to-face contact between teachers and students. The amount of time spent on the actual teaching of an extramural course equals that spent on a similar course at the parent university. The courses are regarded as residential courses, that is the student must attend classes, seminars or tutorials or must utilise the facilities of the multi-sensory learning laboratories and make the usual regular contact with the tutor (or resource person). The majority of extramural courses are provided in the evenings.

Extramural courses have never presented problems to nurse educators. In South Africa we have always believed that extramural degree courses for nurses should be established by all the existing residential universities as and when such facilities are established for other disciplines in satellite towns or in towns in different parts of the country. Extramural courses cannot meet the needs of a whole country, for such courses have to be established in areas where they would be viable. Viability is limited by the numbers of practitioners who live close to the centre and are able to attend evening classes.

What is an external degree? Before the University of South Africa (UNISA) became a teaching university it awarded external degrees to persons who presented themselves for examination but who had not studied at a constituent college of this university. Such university colleges offered internal or residential or extramural study facilities. External students studied on their own. They obtained a curriculum from the university and through private study prepared themselves for examination for an external degree. The degrees were all the same; the method of instruction was the basis for the words residential, extramural or external. These words did not appear on the certificate. The method of tuition was merely indicated on the application for admission to the examination.

In the case of true external degrees or diplomas statutory provision is made for an organisation or institution to award such external degrees or diplomas. Such organisations also present degrees or diplomas to graduates of some tertiary educational institutions which are not universities. It is the function of these organisations to define the broad objectives and curriculum content of such degrees or diplomas and to evaluate competence mastery by a series of examinations. However, the organisation does not participate in any way in the teaching programme or in the self-learning activities of the student.

There are some well-known universities or university systems which provide for their own external degrees or diplomas. The University of London and the University of the State of New York are examples of such organisations.

In South Africa, the South African Nursing Council is a good example of an organisation which in reality provides an external national qualification for nurses at the diploma level.

Teletuition

In South Africa we are fortunate to have a compromise system for studying for degrees or diplomas, namely teletuition. It is this system which provided an answer to the needs and the dilemmas of the nursing profession in South Africa. Strictly speaking, teletution means distance teaching. It can be equated to extramural or off-campus education in that the student is exposed to contact with her lecturers in the subject via the written word, multi-sensory media and occasional decentralised group discussions. Study guides, prescribed and reference books, tutorial letters, prescribed projects, records, films, cassettes, microfiche material, telephones, workshops and preceptors for control of field work all play a part in this system. A direct tutorial relationship between the lecturer and the student is developed. The evaluation system depends not only on year-end examinations, but in borderline cases also on work done during the academic year.

The University of South Africa (UNISA) has introduced several nursing degree courses and an advanced nursing diploma course to meet the needs of nurses in Southern Africa for continuing education. This acceptance of a non-traditional approach to nursing education arises from five very important issues, namely:

(i) the trend of competence-based learning or self-activity learning

(ii) the need for the nursing profession to make continuing education programmes available to its members

(iii) the inability of the majority of nurses to attend residential universities for extended periods

(iv) the availability of multi-sensory media to facilitate the learning process

(v) recognition of the fact that a developed society is judged in terms of the way in which it enables the individual to realise his or her potential to the full.

Let us examine the first two issues briefly before discussing what we are trying to do at UNISA, because these two issues constitute the rationale for the establishment of the new advanced nursing courses at UNISA. The other issues are so self-evident that they need no further discussion.

The competence based self-activity trend in education

Throughout the world the structure of education is changing. This is already affecting nursing education at many levels. One of the most meaningful aspects of the new trend in education is the break with the traditional patterns of teaching. Two main features of this break are that it is essential that learning must take place not only in the halls of learning, but also in the community, and that the traditional role of the teacher must change. No longer must the teacher be a person who bombards the student with a torrent of words in the learning situation. The focus is no longer on the teacher as a teacher, but has shifted to a more meaningful role. In a competence-mastery or self-activity learning situation the teach is a mentor who stands in a tutorial relationship to the student to guide her, to help plan her studies, to act as a guide to learning resources, to clarify concepts to help her to express her thoughts in a concise and logical manner, and to evaluate her competence in the mastery of her subject. The teacher's function is to help the student to avoid obsolescence of knowledge by highlighting the basic reasons for obsolescence, namely that knowledge is lost through lack of use and through the non-acquisition or non-utilisation of new knowledge.

In competence-mastery learning there is no need for every student to be in contact with the tutor at the same time and in the same place to hear the same content. The tutor defines the specific learning objectives and guides the student with regard to the methods to be used and the resources available to her for reaching the objectives. Three concepts dominate this approach, namely:

(i) what a person knows is more important than where, when and how she learned it

(ii) learning objectives should be clearly defined

(iii) valid and reliable methods should be devised to measure the student's knowledge.

Teachers are no longer expected to convey a mass of content detail to groups of passive student recipients, nor to work their nerves to a frazzle trying to make each bit of information interesting to every student in the group. It is no longer the teacher's function to drive her students relentlessly to ensure that as many as possible pass the examinations. The new approach places the responsibility for achieving the required level of mastery of her subject squarely on the student. The teacher is there as a setter of objectives, a resource person, a mentor, a preceptor and an evaluator of performance. This is the system in the non-traditional residential universities, and even in some of the traditional ones.

Why nurse teachers have taken so long to come around to this system of teaching is a mystery. After all, they have known for a very long time that individuals learn in different ways and at different speeds. They have known that students have different styles of learning, and that all students are capable of learning in some way or another. It has taken a long time for them to insist that the responsibility for learning rests primarily with the student, and that the teacher's main responsibility is that of a planner, a facilitator and an evaluator whose task it is to develop the potential of each student rather than to stuff his head full of knowledge which he may resent, or find boring, or be unable to assimilate.

Teletuition is a non-traditional teaching strategy based on modern educational concepts. It is strengthened by the desire of the individual to learn, because it is he or she who seeks out the learning centre and voluntarily exposes himself or herself to its influence. It appears to be a strategy which would meet some of the needs of continuing education for nurses.

Focus on continuing education

The need for continuing education for nurses has been debated at some length at conferences, seminars and professional meetings. Substantial efforts have been made to make annual courses available to as many nurses as possible. For the purpose of this paper we will acknowledge that there is a grave need for continuing education and that the greatest need at this stage is for some formal courses which will serve as foundation courses for further development.

This is necessary because the focal point in continuing education for nurses has now moved beyond the in-service education component. The emphasis goes beyond the identification of deficiencies in the performance of practitioners or in the system of health care. Today continuing education tends to focus on an anticipatory approach, which is directed towards the preparation of workers who will have to organise and administer services and to participate in nursing processes very different from those with which they are currently familiar. Social, economic, cultural, educational, physical, biochemical, psychological, political, philosophical and ideological pressures are shaping a new world which will demand a different system of health care, an unprecedented range and depth of knowledge and preparedness, and extensive knowledge of the implications of intercultural interactions for health practice. The range and extent of the changes that will occur over the next quarter of a century are not known, neither can they be anticipated, although present indications are that such changes will be profound as a result of societal changes and the explosion of scientific knowledge.

How does one cope with such a situation? There are four factors which will play a decisive role in the ability of the nursing profession to provide the type of service that the future demands. Bearing in mind that each tomorrow constitutes the future and today is already the past, there is an urgent need to give attention to these factors. They are the will and the confidence to accept change and not to fear it, for change has always been with mankind; proper scientific preparation in the basic education of the nurse, with particular attention to a sound foundation in the physical, biological, medical, nursing and social sciences; adequate preparation and development of skill in using the scientific method to discover new knowledge; and the development of inquiring, self-reliant minds which are geared to lifelong self-learning.

Health professional competence has four dimensions, namely scientific, technological, societal and personal dimensions. The function of continuing education should be to enable the worker to cope with society's needs in all these dimensions and, in so doing, to contribute to the enrichment of society. A person who masters self-education contributes to society's development in a measure far exceeding such achievements as improvements in service performance or public accountability, which are so often stated to be the aim of continuing education. He or she adds to the intellectual capital of his or her group. Such a person does not fear the future, but makes it and manipulates it for the well-being of society.

The nursing degree courses offered at UNISA

The first nursing degree courses offered at UNISA owe their structure to certain fundamental factors. The development of the health services in South Africa is hampered by the lack of senior nursing personnel with university education beyond the professional registration level. The courses at residential universities cannot meet the need for senior nursing personnel because large numbers of highly competent nurses are for many reasons unable to register at residential universities.

At present 80% of all registered nurses in practice are married. Few of them are able to move to a residential university for one to three years of full-time study. Health service organisations outside the big cities also find it difficult to release personnel for protracted periods of study at residential universities. Many registered nurses retire temporarily from nursing while raising their families. Nevertheless they wish to pursue their studies so that when they return to nursing they will be able to make a worthwhile contribution to the health services. Furthermore, nurses working in the private (profit-making) sector do not receive bursaries or study leave for post-basic education. They have to resign from their posts if they wish to register for such courses. This results in a loss of manpower for a time and also affects their economic status. Many nurses wish to pursue their studies at university level as a means of developing the attitude of mind, the skills and the potential which will help them to keep abreast of the demands of the future.

The introduction of selected nursing degrees and diplomas at non-residential universities became imperative. The teletuition system as conducted by UNISA seems to be the answer to a prayer.

The following pertinent factors were taken into consideration when the Board negotiated with the UNISA authorities for the introduction of the course:

(i) The standard of the various proposed courses *vis-à-vis* other academic courses at UNISA and *vis-à-vis* the courses for nursing degrees at residential universities. In addition, the proposed standards were compared with those for similar courses at American and British universities.

(ii) The need to obtain registration of the qualifications with the South African Nursing Council in more than one professional capacity.

(iii) The need to make the degrees academically strong and to reduce the cost of the proposed qualifications by incorporating relevant existing academic courses into the structure of both the proposed baccalaureate and the diploma courses.

(iv) The needs of the health services for particular categories of personnel and the needs of the greatest number of nurses who would be making use of this system of continuing education.

(v) The number of teaching personnel necessary to start the programme. It was envisaged that a start could be made with one well-qualified, experienced nurse educator, who would initially be assisted by field supervisors who would control practical work. Personnel could be increased as the planning advanced.

(vi) The possible enrolment. It was difficult to predict what the initial enrolment for such courses would be. At the time (1975) approximately 200 nurses were enrolled with UNISA, primarily on social science degree courses. Some 150 nurses indicated that they were anxious to enrol for the proposed nursing courses. However, experience has shown that not all those who show interest in a course enrol for it, and it was envisaged that enrolments for the first year would probably be low until information concerning the courses reached a sufficiently large number of nurses. By October 1975 no less than 700 nurses had enrolled for the first teletuition nursing degrees.

It was decided to start with functional nursing degrees and in due course to examine the possibility of introducing subjects more closely connected with the actual nursing process. It was envisaged that in time such courses would cater for a variety of nurses' continuing education needs. It was also hoped that nursing colleges would eventually be drawn within the ambit of the university on the lines outlined by the Van Wyk and De Vries Commission Report (1973:181-225).

On 1 July 1975 South African nurses made history once more when the Department of Nursing was formally established at the University of South Africa. I was appointed Head of the Department, with a seat on the Senate. It was proposed to register the first students by 15 October 1975. Indications were that the department would grow fairly rapidly, for the nurses of South Africa were reaching out to seize this golden opportunity to secure advanced education in a world-famous university. Nurses are intensely proud of the fact that nursing has taken root in this great university which has done so much to develop the potential of citizens of all races, not only in our own country, but across our borders. The first of July 1975 is indeed a momentous day in nursing history in South Africa, for now university education is within the reach of every registered nurse. I am indeed privileged and blessed to be part of this great historical development. My medical and nursing colleagues see it as the most important part of my life's work in nursing.

The university resolved to introduce a BA (Curationis), an Hons BA (Curationis), an MA (Curationis), a D Litt et Phil and a Diploma in Advanced Nursing Science. The South African Nursing Council had already agreed to register the degrees in their various categories of post-registration education.

Will these courses be of the same high standard as that of nursing degrees at residential universities? This is the question many nurses asked while the Board of the South African Nursing Association was negotiating with the UNISA authorities. Nurses also wished to know whether the introduction of teletuition courses would not detract from the recognition that South African nursing degrees currently enjoy. There was no need to fear on these scores. Among the health professionals in South Africa nurses were the first with an educational innovation of this type, and already other health professionals are showing an interest in this. I predict that one day there will be a faculty of Health Sciences at UNISA which will cater for the needs of all categories of health professional.

The doubting Thomases in the nursing profession can rest assured that the standard of the courses compares very well indeed with courses of a similar nature at residential universities, as well as with non-professional degree courses.

The courses are also available to nurses across the borders of South Africa. They are open to all registered nurses, irrespective of race, colour or creed, provided they are able to cope with either the English or the Afrikaans language. They are provided so that the people of Africa in particular may benefit from the services of knowledgeable health service managers, nurse educators and community health practitioners.

Has teletuition proved beneficial to the nursing profession?

There is ample evidence to indicate that numerous benefits have accrued to the nursing profession as a result of the introduction of teletuition courses. There can be no development in the nursing profession without widespread provision for advanced nursing education. Distance education (teletuition) has contributed enormously to bringing advanced education within reach of all professional nurses. It has many advantages:

(i) It provides university education to large numbers of nurses who would otherwise be deprived of the opportunity to advance in their chosen career.

(ii) It is economical. The nurse contributes to the national economy and to the health care of citizens while she is studying. Compared with conventional nursing education systems, it ensures a less expensive course for the nurse.

(iii) It has greatly increased the number of university graduates in specific fields of nursing and has helped to establish a firm research base for nursing in Southern Africa. It has also contributed to the development of writing skills among nurses. Many nurse authors are now emerging.

(iv) It has enabled a large number of nurses to obtain high academic or executive positions, and has helped South African nurses to take their place in international health matters.

There are many other advantages. The above are merely an indication of the benefits that accrue. The following tables indicate the extent of the contribution made by UNISA to the production of senior nursing personnel.

Table 13.1 The number of registered tutors, nurse administrators and community health nurses on the registers of the SA Nursing Council as at 31 December 1986, and the number of persons in these categories who qualified at UNISA

Category	Total number of persons in these categories on the register Period 1945-1986 = 41 years (1)	Total number of persons in these categories who hold Unisa qualifications Period 1979-1986 = 7 years (2)
Tutor	2 086	615 = 29,5%
Nurse administrator	2 159	988 = 45,8%
Community nurse	5 328	1 367 = 25,7%
Grand total	9 573	2 970 = 31%

(1) Records of the SA Nursing Council C/2 M87 1986
(2) Records of the University of South Africa

The above is a 7-year versus a 41-year output! The contribution of UNISA takes on further meaning when regard is had to the production of these categories of personnel in the year 1976 and the year 1986.

Table 13.2 Registered tutors, nurse administrators and community health nurses produced by university and other tertiary education institutions in the years 1976 and 1986 respectively

Registered category	Year	No produced by other universities and tertiary education institutions	No of participating universities and other tertiary education institutions	No produced by UNISA
Tutor	1976(1)	71	10	–
Nurse administrator		43	8	–
Community health nurse		37	6	–
Tutor	1986(2)	123(53%)	13	109(47%)
Nurse administator		155(49,4%)	11	159(50,6%)
Community health nurse		123(37%)	13	209(63%)

(1) SANC Record 1976 C2/M77
(2) SANC Record 1986 C2/M87 (I&J)

The courses at UNISA started in 1976 and the first degrees and diplomas were awarded in 1979. In the period January 1979 to January 1987 the following degrees and diplomas were awarded to nurses:

Diploma in Advanced Nursing Science	307
BA(Cur)	1 357
Hons BA(Cur)	132
MA(Cur)	25
D Litt et Phil	12
TOTAL	1 833

The first Black nurses to obtain doctorates in South Africa graduated from UNISA, and the first two Black Professors in Nursing are UNISA graduates. Many UNISA graduates proceed overseas to read for a Master's degree. They all do well in their studies.

The contribution to the development of the health services through the development of the nursing profession is self-evident. Distance education in nursing is indispensable in a country such as South Africa. The decade to the end of this century will see it grow from strength to strength. The ethos of nursing in South Africa is being profoundly affected by distance education for nurses. It is not possible to predict what the effect will be by the year 2000 AD.

References

Van Wyk & De Vries Commission. 1973. *Main Report of the Commission of Inquiry into Universities*. Pretoria: Government Printer. (pp 181-225.)
Memorandum on the proposed content of degree and diploma courses in nursing science for possible introduction by the University of South Africa. (Board – SA Nursing Association to Rector, University of South Africa. (6 January 1975.)

General bibliography

American Nurses' Association. 1974. Continuing Education. In *Guidelines for State Nurses' Associations*. Kansas City: ANA.

Commission on Non-traditional Study. 1973. *Diversity of Design*. San Francisco: Jossey Bass.

Cooper, Signe S. 1975. Trends in Continuing Education in the United States. *International Nursing Review*, 22(4-202): 117-120.

Gould, S & Cross, KP. 1933. *Explorations in Non-traditional Study*. San Francisco: Jossey Bass.

14

New perspectives on nursing education in the Republic of South Africa

Introductory commentary

There is a great deal of uncertainty among nurses, hospital administrators and medical practitioners about contemporary developments in nursing education. There is evidence of mental stagnation on this issue. The result is a tendency to thwart developments, to decry their value and to predict total disaster for the nursing education system and the nursing services. Such issues as the freezing of student posts, other financial restraints, misuse of nursing students, disregard for their learning needs and dissatisfaction among the ranks of students are overlooked. All the ills are attributed to changing perspectives in nursing education. Only the future will show whether contemporary thought on nursing education is valid in the South African context. Stout hearts are necessary to implement and guide new developments.

THE ADDRESS

Introduction

'There is a tide in the affairs of man,
which taken at the flood, leads on to fortune;
Omitted, all the voyage of their life.
Is bound in shallows and miseries.
On such a full sea are we now afloat,
And we must take the current when it serves,
Or lose our ventures.'

Julius Caesar IV iii

Such a moment for decision and action has come for nursing in South Africa. What nursing is to become in the last decades of this century, its nature in the incoming years of the 21st century, and what contribution it will be able to make to the health care of the peoples of Southern Africa will depend on how nurse planners, managers, educators and the profession at large face the challenge confronting the profession.

Will the profession, like a Canute of old, tell the mighty sea to roll back and not wet the royal feet, or will it breast the tide of opportunity to become master of the sea of problems threatening to engulf it? Will it set sail with the floodtide, or will it be left stranded on desolate beaches? This is the million dollar question that must be answered by the profession this year. Next year it may be too late to find satisfactory answers.

Nursing resources will be strained

The challenge of the next few years will tax nursing resources, ingenuity, competence and commitment to the utmost. At a conservative estimate, the total population will be approximately 46 631 000 by the year 2000. This is a projected increase of 22 777 000 persons in two decades (Scientific Report 1983: 124, 127, 130, 132). Coupled with this enormous increase in population are such social and economic issuses as:

(i) a further slowing of the economic growth of the community

(ii) desertification of a large part of the country due to prolonged and frequent droughts, resulting in increased rural poverty and depopulation of the rural areas

(iii) an accelerated trend in urbanisation due to social, political and economic causes

(iv) increased awareness of the benefits of modern health practices and a greater demand for more extensive and improved health services

(v) increased membership among Black and Coloured persons of medical aid schemes

(vi) expansion of both institutional and non-institutional health services by the state and the private sector.

All this will strain the financial and human resources of this country to the utmost.

The heavy burden of maintaining the already existing sophisticated hospitals maintained by the state in urban areas will have to be lightened by the expansion of domiciliary care, clinics, day hospitals and hostel services for non-acutely ill persons who require some degree of hospitalisation. Increased membership of medical aid schemes will lead to greater privatisation of the health services.

All this will require more and better prepared nurses, who are able to:

(i) define their professional roles

(ii) help formulate and implement health care policies

(iii) take on leadership roles

(iv) do much-needed research

(v) participate in the education of the public and the profession at both basic and post-registration levels

(vi) understand and explain the rationale of their ethical code and concepts and the theory of their professional practice

(vii) practise their profession with knowledge, insight, skill, compassion and concern for the human beings at the receiving end

(viii) fulfil a collegial role in the health team.

It is estimated that in order to cope the nursing education system should produce some 36 000 additional registered nurses by the turn of this century. A more realistic figure would be 20 000. These nurses must be able to provide a comprehensive health care service and must meet the criteria listed in the preceding paragraph. If they cannot meet these requirements, their professional preparation is at fault.

Cost of producing the modern nursing force

The production of these nurses will cost millions. At the same time, the infrastructure for healthy living demands the provision of housing, water, sanitation, lighting, employment, transport facilities, education and welfare benefits at an increasing rate. The economic resources of South Africa will be strained to the limit. The most difficult task of all will be to provide a health service within the constraints of a limited national budget.

Cost of health care

In 1980 the cost of health care in South Africa and the national states amounted to R2 737 037 387, whereas the Gross National Product (GNP) in that year was R59 279 000 000. Thus no less than 4,6% of the GNP was spent on health. South Africa is only partly a developed country. The cost of developing the country to full first world status will multiply many, many times in the next two decades, and health care costs will escalate accordingly. Every provider of essential services therefore has a major task to ensure that health care costs are kept within the financial resources of the community and that all the care that is provided is cost-effective. It is the health professional working within a realistic health care policy who will determine the size of the nation's health bill, for his or her guidance must assist in the elimination of those socio-economic and environmental issues that are basic to the erosion of the health status of individuals and of the community. The profession cannot deliver the kind of service that is envisaged, and indeed expected of it, if it clings to outdated methods, takes refuge in clichés, blinkers its vision with outdated customs and prejudice, and hobbles its performance with ritualistic approaches and methods of a bygone era.

The nurse who has to function within a comprehensive health care system must be educated and trained in a comprehensive manner. If we were to abide by the traditional methods of educating nurses it would take six years to produce a comprehensive prepared nurse, and she would have received this education as a non-integrated, piece-meal process and be primarily hospital orientated in her outlook instead of 'comprehensive' orientated, or 'psycho-social-somatic-institutional-non-institutional-individual-family-and-community orientated'.

The profession will be unable to meet the challenges inherent in the problems bedevilling the closing years of this century if it clings to a nursing education system that has not kept pace with the social, educational and health developments of the age in which we live. Renewal is urgently necessary. All contemporary professions are facing the same need for renewal as the nursing profession.

Tidal wave of change

The nursing profession is confronting a tidal wave of change. Will it take the tide at the flood and make a further and even more indelible mark on the history of social development in South Africa than it has done up to now? Let us see why I believe that the nursing profession in this country will, despite the prognostications of the prophets of doom, write another glorious chapter in the history of our profession and in the social history of our country. I want to take you back a century, and to ask you whether the nurses of this country have not succeeded against almost insurmountable odds to build the profession that we know today.

Problems faced by the pioneers of professional nursing in South Africa

It is fitting here to look back to the problems encountered by the founders of professional nursing in South Africa. A century ago Sister Henrietta Stockdale and her very small band of pioneers faced many problems similar to those confronting nursing in the latter part of the 20th century. I believe their task was far more formidable than ours.

Let us examine the similarities between their position and ours:

(i) Their number was out of proportion to the population that had to be served. Indeed their number was pitiably small.

(ii) They had to cope with the problems arising from a diversity of cultures, languages and political viewpoints, and with an extremely rapidly growing population.

(iii) They had to cope with a changing constitutional and political situation.

(iv) They had to provide a health service throughout the length and breadth of South Africa and had to do so with the minimum of resources. There being a shortage of doctors and pharmacists, and a marked maldistribution of such personnel, nurses had to go where other health professionals declined to go. They had to lay the foundations of hospital services and domiciliary nursing services, as well as of private practitioner nursing services. When the need arose they had to provide whatever 'medical' care they could as an emergency measure, and had to dispense medicines as well. In the case of acute illness they had to get the patient to a doctor or hospital. This had to be done despite the fact that telephones were very few and far between, the motor car was not yet in use, train services were irregular, roads were almost impassable, and hospitals and doctors were located in remote towns. Removal of a patient to a distant hospital under such circumstances was fraught with danger. It was, in fact, a life-threatening situation. Consequently the nurse did what she could and kept the patient at home. If she could not obtain the services of a doctor, as was invariably the case, she did her best for the patient and trusted to God's help, her devotion, her professional knowledge and her mother-wit to see her and her patient through the situation. She was an expert at involving the family in the decision-making and care process.

(v) They had to provide health care in unhygienic, disorganised mining camps, on lonely farms, in scattered villages, in malaria-ridden outposts, and in small, ill-equipped cottage hospitals. The threat of war and economic disaster was ever-present.

(vi) They had to provide comprehensive nursing care, coping with all general physical and mental health problems, infectious diseases, and domiciliary nursing and midwifery. They did so in a unified manner. Because there were so few of them they had to do everything that required some form of health care assistance. Wherever they served the health of the population improved. The benefits of modern medical science and modern approaches to health care were carried to distant villages and towns, to lonely farms and remote mission stations. They were the first to propose that the patient, his family and the community should make an input into the health care of the individual and his group. Realism, because of the extent of the health care problem, nurtured this concept. It is a post-World War II phenomenon that the state is expected to provide for all the health care needs of society, without society making an effort to keep its members healthy or to contribute to the care of those who suffer a breakdown in or an impediment to health.

(vii) They recognised the need for a professional code of practice and for ethical concepts that were relevant to the needs of a developing country and a developing profession.

(viii) They recognised the need for legal recognition of the profession of nursing, and thus obtained statutory recognition of the profession. They ensured that the nurse in South Africa was legally recognised as a practitioner, with all the rights and duties this entailed, before this was achieved anywhere else in the world.

(ix) They had to develop a nursing education system to provide much-needed nursing personnel. They had to do so with scarce resources and had to follow uncharted paths to reach their objectives. They were short of teachers, of nurses and of preceptors who could serve as role models. They had little money for their educational task and had to develop a new category of professional person who could stand shoulder to shoulder with the doctor in the fight to bring health to the people of South Africa. Their resources were limited, but their enthusiasm and faith were boundless.

(x) The aim of their nursing education was to provide well-trained personnel as rapidly as possible to meet the growing demand for nurses. The quality of the nursing education was a key issue, for this contributed to the quality of care provided by ward sisters, district nurses, private duty nurses, matrons and midwives. Careful selection of students, a pervasive philosophy of service, a deep sense of ethical values and of personal and professional commitment, responsibility and accountability characterised their educational endeavours. The concept of situational analysis in planning a training programme is evident in the first educational programme they produced, thereby giving nursing education in this part of the world a national character despite the fact that it was modelled on the Nightingale System.

(xi) Once professional registration was accomplished and the professional practice status of the nurse was assured, they realised that the education of professional practitioners needed to be conducted within a system of higher education. It was for this reason that Sister Henrietta wanted nursing education to be placed under the auspices of the Department of Education of the Colony of the Cape of Good Hope. She wanted nursing education to be placed on the same level as the education of teachers for the primary and secondary education system and to be financed from the resources of the taxpayer. She saw nursing education as being on a par with teacher education. She saw the practical dimension of nurse training as 'pupilage' and not as work, even though nurses provided patient care during the learning period. 'Pupilage' was already in force in teacher education. She was well ahead of her time in this respect. Today we would speak about 'learning experiences under the supervision of a preceptor'. The concept is the same.

It is interesting to recall that the nursing education system of the then Colony of the Cape of Good Hope was the first in the world to enter its students for an external statutory examination. This was the examination of the Colonial Medical Council of the Cape of Good Hope and was a professional examination. From the beginning of nursing education in this country the concept of statutory examinations at the hands of a statutory authority was entrenched. The present process of decentralisation of examinations retains this concept that an external statutory authority (the university) should have the final decision in the examination process, while enabling the teachers who have prepared the future practitioners to have a major share in the final evaluation of the students' competence to practice.

Nursing education as part of the post-secondary education system

Sister Henrietta's ideal that nursing education should form part of the post-secondary education system of the country on a par with teacher education has remained with the nurses of this country. Its implementation has been delayed for six main reasons which are dealt with in the paragraphs which follow.

Adverse social conditions

Serious social conditions pertained in the country for several decades after the turn of the 19th century. Three devastating wars occurred. The South African War (1899-1902), with its incredible aftermath of poverty, social disorganisation and political bitterness, ushered in the 20th century. World War I (1914-1918) and its huge cost to an impoverished agricultural nation crippled the economy. World War II (1939-1945) brought industrialisation, an extensive urban drift of Black workers and their families, and a large national debt. Droughts and depression weakened the economy, which had to be revitalised and industrialised.

Nurses carried the burden of providing health care at low cost

During the difficult years between 1904 and 1944 the nursing education system provided health services at low cost. The concept of the student as the main component of the hospital work force became entrenched. Health authorities were loath to change this system.

Statutory control by South African Medical Council a constraint

Progress was not possible until the statutory control of nursing education was taken away from the South African Medical Council and vested in the South African Nursing Council.

Shortcomings of the secondary education system a barrier to the development of nursing education

The secondary school system could not produce the number of students with their senior certificate or matriculation that the profession required for admission to their courses. Nursing required extensive intakes of students to provide the work force needed to maintain the expanding hospital services at a relatively low cost. The profession had to compromise on admission requirements to meet societal needs. In doing so it dealt nursing education a serious blow.

Overseas training for nurse educators a major constraint

Tutors had to be educated in Great Britain until the South African universities could undertake this responsibility. The attitude of many senior nurses delayed development, since many of them believed that a high level of tutor education could be obtained only in Great Britain. This limited numbers and delayed progress.

Attitude of some senior members of the profession a major constraint

Between 1944 and 1984 the attitude of many senior members of the profession impeded progress. This was mainly due to the fact that they saw students as the main component of the work force, because the principle of service for education instead of education for service had become firmly entrenched.

Heritage of the pioneers

The pioneers of the period 1876 to 1944 made an unprecedented contribution to the social development of South Africa, and in particular to the development of its health services. They left a rich heritage of ethical values, a sound philosophy of service, courage and devotion to duty. Above all, they left this generation of nurses with the following:

(i) The concept that nurses have to meet the challenge of their times in order to provide for the health of the nation. Whenever a doctor is not available the nurse must do whatever she can to meet the patient's nursing and medical needs. This became 'nursing' in South Africa. Nurses served in lonely and dangerous outposts and trekked over desolate country which lacked transport services to bring their healing mission to the people of this country.

(ii) An educational system and an educational ideal which could evolve into the pattern that is being developed at present.

(iii) A professional practice system which could be adjusted to meet the demands of the times.

(iv) Awareness of the need for professional solidarity within a professional association.

Each generation of pioneers passed its vision on to the next generation, and each generation laid more bricks to build the great edifice that is modern South African nursing. Each one of us in this room owes part of what we are to our predecessors.

Winds of change

At present the winds of social change in our country are buffeting us about. Today we are the pioneers of the new systems necessary to meet the health needs of our country. Are not the problems that we are facing today of the same type as those that our predecessors faced when they laid the foundations of professional nursing in South Africa? The problems we face are similar to those faced by the pioneers of the last century. They succeeded in the face of great odds. Let us ask ourselves whether we have less courage, less vision, less ability and less determination than our predecessors possessed? Do we have a lower level of awareness of human need than they possessed? Did they have a greater sense of professional responsibility and a keener philosophy of service than we cherish? Did they have a greater will to succeed on behalf of the nation than we have today? Only the future can confirm or deny this. I believe that all the great qualities that our pioneers possessed are present in abundance in this generation of nurses. They too can overcome the obstacles. They too have the ability to identify needs, and the knowhow and the sense of commitment to meet them.

I believe we can build as they built, toil as they toiled, and leave as proud a record of service as they left. They took nursing in South Africa into the 20th century and laid the foundations upon which successive generations have been able to build. They showed us how to meet changing needs, how to adapt to the demands of the times. Will our successors one hundred years from now say of us what I am saying now about the nurses who made the nursing profession in this country great during the last one hundred years? I say 'they built better than they knew. If you seek their monument, look around you' (*si monumentum quaeris circumspice*).

Nursing colleges and universities must recognise the challenge of the times

I am confident that all nursing education institutions will recognise the challenge of our times and take careful note of:

(i) the ever-expanding role of the nurse

(ii) the increasingly comprehensive nature of her work, whether at sophisticated specialist level or at home care level

(iii) the scarcity of financial resources and the social onslaught from within and without the profession on our philosophy and value systems and on the nature of our services.

The challenge

The provision of health services will provide the profession with great challenges, the main one being the education of nurses at the basic level. If the basic level of nursing education is geared towards community needs, contemporary educational thought and the provision of a comprehensive foundation of knowledge which will serve as the basis for advanced formal education as well as for lifelong learning, we will provide a sound professional education. The provision of knowledgeable, responsible, accountable, creative, thinking practitioners must be the focus of all the efforts we make to meet the health needs of our country. The future lies in the hands of the nurse educators of today.

The need for a positive contribution from nurse educators

I believe that nurse educators must break with the customs of the past, not only in the way they approach their subject content, but in their approach to the system of nursing education as a whole, for in their hands lies the production of the persons who have to lead the profession and to provide the services.

There may be some overt, and a considerable degree of covert, resistance to the new approach to the preparation of nurse practitioners. Of course it will be hard to accept that we did not do the right thing when we required a three-year period of training for general nursing, a one-year period for midwifery, a one-year period for psychiatric nursing and a one-year period for community nursing. No less than six years' training for the content of a four-year course! Whatever made us do this?

Let us never forget that this pattern was forced on nursing education through the division of responsibility for the health services and not as a result of an educational rationale. It became entrenched because the nursing education system was based on hospitals and was not located in post-secondary educational institutions.

Our problems with nursing education and its location within the post-secondary education system arise from the constitutional history of our country, which was at one time part of a colonial system. This system bequeathed to us a tradition of division of responsibility for health services, and of hospital-based nursing education. This tradition emanated from the mother country, Great Britain, at a time when that country had a system of divided health services and a system of nursing education which provided its numerous infirmaries with a cheap work force. It was not an educational concept or ideal, but the vision of a cheap source of labour that dominated the scene. As a result of this influence student nurses, in the sacred name of education, have given this country many thousands of man years of service in return for education. It was service for education before education for service, which took a secondary place.

The need for a break with tradition

The long-established tradition that the nursing service director is also the head of the nursing school will require a revolutionary change in thinking. She will now assume a new role as a member of a college council which is the governing authority of a nursing college. In this role she will be concerned with the educational needs of the student and *not* with the staffing needs of her service.

Urgent problems to be faced

It is not only the nursing service manager who will have to do some new thinking. I believe that the problems most urgently requiring attention are the following:
  (i) The preparation and/or updating of nurse educators and nurse plan-
      ners to enable them to prepare future nurse practitioners in a truly

comprehensive manner, with horizontal and vertical integration of subject matter, while ensuring that their foundation in each subject is firm and adequate to their practice needs as well as providing a basis for further education and for the crediting of courses in related fields of study.

(ii) The need for nurse educators to acknowledge that they must be able to:

   – identify the learning experiences and knowledge base essential for contemporary professional practice
   – devise modern teaching strategies
   – identify the parameters, intricacies and legal dimensions of professional practice
   – breathe life into the clay of a curriculum and make it a vibrant, living thing
   – imbue the student with a sense of professionalism, the value of her role in society, the importance of nursing philosophy and nursing values, the importance of professional socialisation and the dilemmas of contemporary ethical issues in health care.

(iii) The need for nurse educators to regain their clinical proficiency and to become part of the teaching team in the clinical situation.

(iv) The need for nurse educators to develop their own academic and social abilities.

(v) The need for nurse educators to re-focus their sights on patients and students rather than on methods of teaching.

Competent nurse practitioners to be prepared

Nurse educators have to prepare nurses to be competent nurse practitioners capable of functioning effectively in institutional (state and private), community health and private practice services.

Books and articles refer to such newly registered nurse practitioners as 'first level' registered nurses, whatever that may mean. This is a debatable viewpoint. The South African Nursing Council requires a student nurse to be prepared so that on registration she is able to cope with the nursing needs of man from before birth to death at an advanced age, and to do so in the general, psychiatric, community health and midwifery fields for all those health conditions that occur as a constant factor in the South Africa community. This does not imply that she must be able to cope with the highly complex (and statistically less frequent) conditions that are treated in some highly specialised departments of large, academic central hospitals. The South African Nursing Council requires a newly registered nurse to be able to provide nursing care in promotive, preventive, curative and rehabilitative health care situations, and to be able to do so on an integrative basis within the social, economic and cultural context of her patients/clients. She must be able to function as an 'advocate' of the patient to present his case to the health team, the health care situation and the community. She must function on a collegial basis with other members of the health team, either at close contact level or 'distance practice' level. Above all, she must be able to function as the professional partner of the doctor in the health care process, for the patient is her patient as much as he is the doctor's patient.

Such concepts as nursing diagnosis, prescribing a nursing regimen, the treatment and care of the individual with health problems, the nature and quality of nursing intervention, determining the value of a health regimen, coordination of activities, advocacy for the patient, the scope and practice of nursing, lifelong learning responsibility, accountability and collegial relationships will be an integral part of the practice of a newly qualified nurse. Therefore she must understand such concepts and be able to implement them as a competent professional practitioner.

The quality of educators will be decisive

This demanding preparation requires knowledgeable, highly skilled and motivated educators who will see each subject and each learning opportunity as a tool to be used for the growth and development and the professional blossoming of the neophyte, and who will see the potential of each student nurse and help her to attain this. Preceptors who are true role models, capable of ensuring that high quality humane scientific care is provided at all times and of interpreting the profession and its aims, as well as society's need for competent caring nurses to the student, are essential. Their contribution will be decisive. Will we produce practitioners with the 'handmaiden' mentality, professionals with the ability to think critically, to act with judgement, knowledge and skill, and to function in a collegial relationship with other members of the health team.

The nurse educator must be able to challenge established concepts and 'clichés'

Many nurse educators talk glibly about providing 'total patient care'. Have they ever challenged this concept? When analysed socio-logically, this phraseology does not make sense. We all use this terminology habitually because for the past 30 years overseas nursing literature has stressed it. It implies that a nurse must supply the total psycho-social-physical needs of her patient in the care situation. Why do we talk such nonsense? From a sociological point of view the health worker is always in a secondary relationship with her patient or client. It is a well-accepted sociological fact that individuals in any secondary relationship share only a part of themselves with others. They do not relate with the 'whole' person, but only with those aspects which are directly concerned with the secondary relationship, and then only in part. This happens even in a primary relationship.

A health client/patient is involved with hospital staff and with other patients. He always protects those aspects which constitute a truly integral part of his life, such as his personal loyalties, his religious and deep-seated cultural beliefs, his feelings and his fears. Every human being, and hence every patient, is really isolated from others to a certain extent. It is part of his individualism. He is never a 'total entity' to others.

The nurse-patient relationship does not constitute a primary relationship, but is always a secondary relationship. While the nurse can never provide 'total' care, she has a duty to see man as a unique individual, to respect his dignity and his rights, to relieve the stresses of the health care situation and of the period of ill-health and to help him maintain his place within his primary relationship. She has a duty to ensure that his care is not dehumanised, that her approach is flexible and responsible, and that his worries are lessened to the extent that this is possible. But let us not talk about 'total' care. I prefer 'comprehensive care', because the psycho-social-physical dimensions of care need to be integrated to bring compassionate, competent health care to the patient in the hands of diverse members of the health team.

We should not teach in 'clichés', but should analyse meaning within the context of the sociological and cultural parameters of nursing in this country. Then, and only then, will we develop a truly South African theory and practice of nursing.

Similarly, we should analyse the concepts 'medical model' and 'nursing model' in a South African, and indeed African, context. Professional nursing in South Africa evolved out of the Nightingale pattern of nursing, the essence of which was to produce nurses to manage nursing care provided by others. Make a careful study of nursing history in the late Victorian era and test this statement of mine! Yet here on the Diamond Fields of South Africa human need gave birth to a system of nursing which was, still is, and will be in the future, essentially a blend of the so-called medical and nursing models. From the very earliest days of professional nursing in this country medicine and nursing moved up and down the health care continuum, constantly overlapping. Harsh reality has always demanded that the nurse must understand the aetiology and manifestations of disease (or health deviation) and diagnosis and therapeutic intervention. To the knowledgeable and concerned doctor and the knowledgeable and concerned nurse, therapeutic intervention means medical and nursing diagnosis and the prescription and implementation of medical treatment and nursing care. These functions complement each other. There is really no such thing as a 'medical' or a 'nursing' model. There is, however, a 'health care model' with major medical and nursing inputs. Let us analyse critically what the literature presents, and let us ask ourselves whether, because our role is so different, our legal status so much more secure, the nature of our education and training so different from that pertaining in the Americas, we are being truly scientific in swallowing overseas concepts 'holus bolus'. I am beginning to question whether all this emphasis on the medical and the nursing model is not perhaps a defensive mechanism developed by teachers who never lay hands on a patient or are never confronted with the diverse health needs of human beings who must receive health care. If one is confronted with actual patient care and patient needs, one finds that there is only 'a health care' model, which is a blend of the two models we are trying so hard to keep apart.

We have to get our perspectives right, not only with regard to our role, the needs of our country, the educational content and strategies of our courses, the philosophy and ethics of our profession and the nature of our practice, but also with regard to the nature of nursing in this part of the world. We have a duty to ensure that nursing on the subcontinent of Africa develops a truly Southern African character and does not become a carbon copy of nursing designed to serve the needs of a different country with different social, cultural, legal and role parameters.

I think the real issues confronting us are not the so-called medical and nursing models, but the fact that, as Alice Blaumgart (1981) says:

the majority of practising nurses today are ill-prepared for a future in which health care for all is the operating premise. Cultural and structural factors in many countries have favoured the retention of a model of nursing education and nursing practice which is firmly tied to hospitals and the perspectives of curative medicine.

Should not our perspectives be directed away from 'the hospital model' of nursing education and from 'the curative model' of nursing practice towards a 'comprehensive health care model' and a comprehensive system of nursing education which has all the legal attributes and characteristics of post-secondary education? I can never associate myself with the senseless enmity of nurses towards doctors which characterises much of the nursing literature from certain parts of the world. It was not nurses who discovered comprehensive health care, although some nurses appear to think this was the case. Preventive and promotive health concepts are as old as medicine itself. The comprehensive health care concept in its modern context is the brainchild of doctors in the public health movement. Of course there are doctors, as there are nurses, who do not understand the concept and do not believe in it.

Students must become responsible and accountable practitioners

The essence of professionalism and of professionhood lies in awareness and observance of responsible and accountable practice. A good nursing education programme leads the student to an awareness that it is not fear of retribution for professional neglect or malpractice that should guide her practice, but concern for the well-being and feelings of her patient/client, for if this is ever-present then medico-legal hazards will be few and far between. Professional recognition from the public and from one's peer group is based on the quality of one's practice and of one's personal and professional behaviour, and on the regard one cherishes for the collective good name of one's profession.

The questions nurse educators must ask themselves

In this new deal for nursing education each nurse educator must ask herself these questions: 'Am I producing a proficient practitioner who will be able to practise confidently and collegially as a member of the modern health team? Will she be able to see her role as a promoter of health irrespective of her field of professional practice? Will she be able to apply the knowledge and techniques of prevention and health promotion and not only those of cure and rehabilitation? Will she be a competent and worthy professional who realises that learning is a lifelong process? Will she be a worthy and compassionate citizen, an asset to the nation, a servant to mankind and a blessing sent by the Almighty to heal and comfort mankind in his hour of need?'

The future is in our own hands

The nursing profession has struggled for close on a century to achieve the role it has today and the professional educational opportunities which are now available. At long last nursing education is recognised as one of the major post-secondary academic systems in this country, and the role of the nurse as the main provider of health care and as the kingpin in the health care system is well and truly established and recognised by the highest health authorities in this country. Our future is in our own hands. How we ride the flood tide of opportunity will depend on whether we go forward as a powerful, useful, respected profession, or prove to be unequal to the task and fail to meet the great expectations of the state and society in general.

Self-preparation for the enormous task at hand, including renewal of philosophy, commitment and direction, is essential. The perspectives for the future are grim if we fail in this task.

Like the pioneers of the last century we are confronted with an unprecedented health care and professional educational task. They tackled it with confidence, and so must we. I believe in the profession and its future. I know we will succeed!

References

Blaumgart, A. 1981. Nursing for a new century – a future framework. *Journal of Advanced Nursing*, 7(1). Blackwell Scientific.

Chaska, NL. 1983. *The nursing profession: a time to speak*. New York: McGraw-Hill.

Davis, CK. 1983. Nursing and the health care debates. *Image: The Journal of Nursing Scholarship*, XV (3).

Kriekemans, A. 1978. *Beschouwinge over een vergeten opvatting van de fundamentele pedagogiek; de christelike appellatiewe pedagogiek*. Antwerpen: Feestrede.

Mauksch, I & Miller, MH. 1981. *Implementing change in nursing*. St Louis: CV Mosby.

Nationaal Verband der KV Verpleegkundigen. 1981. *Verpleegkundigen en gemeenschapszorg*. N. 3 Brussel.

Scientific Report of the President's Council. 1983. Pretoria: Government Printer.

Styles, ML. 1982. *On nursing. Toward a new endowment*. St Louis: CV Mosby.

SANC. 1984. *Discussions on future trends in nursing education*. April 1979-March 1984.

WHO. 1981. *Global strategy for health for all by the year 2000*. Geneva: WHO.

Comments on educational concepts relevant to this section and their significance for the development of the South African ethos of nursing

The ethos of nursing in South Africa has been shaped by many factors. The influence of the diversity of the politico-socio-economic-cultural-religious structure of society on the development of the ethos of nursing as it is perceived in South Africa has been profound. Within the complexity of this total social milieu and the diversity of the health care system, the nursing profession itself has made the major contribution to the development of the South African nursing ethos.

Through the nature of their service, the scope of their practice and the quality of the leaders emerging from their ranks, nurses of all categories have shaped what is understood as the South African nursing ethos, social constraints and opportunities alike being incorporated in its building blocks. This is the trend worldwide.

Constraints such as routinised, rule-by-regulation administration, the stereotyped organisation of services, emphasis on power *over* instead of *with* and distance between leader and led inhibit the development of individuals and the profession as a whole and thus have a negative effect on the shaping of the ethos of nursing. A similar influence is exerted by classroom-bound nurse educators who teach in a lecture-dominated educational system, who view clinical practice as 'demonstrations of procedures' and who do not relate the nursing curriculum to national and local health needs. On the other hand, enlightened, confident nurse administrators who do not fear cooperative management, who are convincing advocates for their patients and personnel, whose work is characterised by understanding of the human beings they serve and the broader needs of the society of which they are a part, and who are able to work in harmony with all the other members of the health team, have a powerful impact on the development of the nursing ethos.

Nurse educators at university, college or clinical area level have great potential to influence the ethos of their profession. The role of the nurse academic and the challenge of the new approach to nursing education in South Africa are highlighted in this section. Chapter 4 in Part 2 deals with the training of nurses for management and the attention of nurse educators is drawn to it.

Through her preparation of student nurses at basic and post-registration level the nurse educator lays the foundations for nursing management. One of the nurse educator's functions is to produce nurse managers, whether by acting as a mentor or through formal teaching. Somebody trained nurse managers in the past – usually those in supervisory positions. However, since the 1950's there has been formal education in managing nursing services. This is provided mainly by nurse educators, whose influence must never be underestimated.

The integration of curriculum content is not readily understood by all, and nurse educators will have to develop a holistic approach with regard to teaching methods if they wish to implement a comprehensive, integrated system of basic nursing education successfully. They cannot allow themselves to think of their students as shut off from the influences of other subjects, their families and their communities.

The prevention of disease and community participation in the provision of health care will never be achieved while educators see their output in individualistic terms as far as both the nature of the disease and the recipient of the care are concerned.

Ill-health forms a vast network – no health syndrome manifesting in the human body leaves the rest of the body unaffected. Similarly, an individual's health status affects his social status. Therefore it is not very fruitful to compartmentalise our teaching into either body systems or disease entities and not integrate other systems into it. The effects of illness on all systems and on the psycho-social milieu must be studied.

Of course, emphasis on a particular aspect of a health problem in a particular individual is due to our training in the natural sciences, where a small area is studied intensively. One has only to listen to nurse educators' arguments about the teaching of anatomy to appreciate that the isolation of a small area of study is a naturalistic approach. What is happening is that nurse educators are carrying such an approach into the social sciences, for health care is fundamentally the study of a social system and human needs. In the comprehensive, integrated approach to nursing education the emphasis is on the interrelationship between facts, phenomena and actions for solving problems.

Illness and health care must be studied in its total context, which includes the psycho-social milieu. The constant factor affecting the needs of the body, the influence of ill-health on the body, the needs of the individual and his family and the individual's social milieu, is interdependence – not just interrelationship. There is interdependence at all levels – between the elements of the physiological body network and those of the social network and between the health team and the social administration network. Credible teaching is teaching which can provide evidence that the interrelatedness of the components of the human health care approach has been fully understood.

The real challenge contained in chapter 14 (New perspectives on nursing education in the Republic of South Africa) lies in the interrelatedness and interdependence of everything the student has to learn. Nurse educators have to take the lead in adopting a holistic approach to health care and must help both basic and post-registration students to think holistically. These students will be the main providers of health care in the years ahead and therefore must understand 'networking' within the human body, the social system, the health care system and the grassroots social engineering systems.

By the year 2000 the products of the new nursing education system will be at the helm of the nursing system in this country. Both they and their nurse educators and mentors will be judged in terms of their output and understanding of comprehensive, integrated health care delivery. The question to be answered will be: have these nurse educators added a new dimension to the ethos of nursing in this country, and do all nurses, irrespective of their posts, see themselves as educators? Do they believe that 'the nurse is a teacher, a teacher, a teacher', for this concept is inherent in the present ethos of nursing.

PART

7

Nursing theories

15

Nursing theories: what is our commitment?*

[Opening address at the Nursing Theories Symposium,
Potchefstroom University for Christian Higher Education,
September 1987]

Introductory commentary

The discipline nursing requires a theoretical foundation. Part of the image of nursing derives from the theoretical framework which determines a particular perspective on nursing. Definitions of nursing reflect social influences and the thinking of the profession about its role in society. The theoretical framework focuses on the patient within his physiological and social milieu as the centre of concern.

There are many theories of nursing. These have developed as the scope of practice of the nurse has broadened and a better understanding of the patient's place in the health care situation has been attained.

The South African Nursing Council's view that nursing is a humanistic science categorises it as a social science. It is concerned with man as a whole, in sickness and in health, within his social system, namely his family, community and society as a whole.

There are many theories of nursing. It would be very restrictive if this were not so, for nursing is a component of the network that is society and societies differ in many ways. Also, the state of the art and science varies from society to society, particularly where there is a surplus of medical practitioners.

Theories provide the body of knowledge necessary for practice and further research. Theory forms the foundation for the nursing process, which is, after all, only a systematic approach to the provision of nursing care based on the scientific method, scientific inquiry and a problem-solving approach and methods. Today nursing must be seen as an interrelationship between art and science, service to mankind being its aim.

The word 'theory' derives from the Greek word *theoria*, which means vision and implies abstract thought. When developing a series of theories to be used pluralistically a nurse educator must think broadly to find a dimension of nursing which will generate concepts for theory construction. The validity of the theories must be researched, as must the need for pluralism in the use of theories.

It would be interesting to examine the philosophy and the actual nursing functions and acts which have existed since the first record of man's activities. It is relatively easy to construct the theory of nursing which existed in early Christian times, or as it emerges from the writings of Florence Nightingale.

Exciting research, intellectual challenges and dialogue with others involved in theory construction lies ahead for this generation of nurses. The challenges are immense, but the rewards will be great. The question is: are we committed to the development of nursing theories which will be meaningful to a country that is part first and part third world, a country in which nursing is a great equaliser?

I am no theorist. My own theory of nursing goes beyond those expounded by the well-known theorists. Because it is the result of empirical observation and

* First published in *Nursing RSA*, February/March 1988.

not of research, it is not relevant in this context, but it has formed the framework for my life's work.

Now it is over to the younger generation!

THE ADDRESS

Introduction

Although there is a wealth of philosophical and even meta-theoretical discussion in South Africa about the phenomenon 'nursing', there is very little evidence of substantive theory building.

In this country the concept nursing as a discipline derives primarily from the following:

(i) Henrietta Stockdale's ideational-idealistic-philosophical approach to what nursing is and the influence of this philosophy on the legislature and on successive generations of nurse educators.

(ii) The wealth of concepts generated by legislation and the actions and pronouncements of the peer group control body, the professional association and the committee which examined nursing's claim to be a science and decided that nursing as a discipline with a preventive, promotive, curative and rehabilitative role parallel to medicine, in addition to its carative role, justified a designation of its own which demonstrates in both the official languages of this country precisely what the concept implies. The Latin 'Curationis', which designates nursing in this country, spells out the wide range of concepts embodied in the words 'nursing' and 'verpleging'.

(iii) The empirical evidence about *what* nursing is doing, *why, when* and *where* it is being done, and *how* and by *whom* it is done.

I reiterate that despite all the intellectual effort expanded on the profession's growth and development, particularly its academic growth and practice dimensions, there is little evidence of substantive theory building. It is for this reason that the Department of Nursing Science and the Bureau for Continuing Education at this university are to be congratulated on their initiative in organising a workshop and a symposium on such a theme.

There are cogent reasons why theory building in this part of the world is in the doldrums. These cannot be wished away and will be with us for a long time. In spite of this we have to have the courage to embark on our voyage of exploration. If we do not start we will never reach a goal.

Let us examine briefly what some of these reasons are, for by careful selection and preparation of nurse educators we may by-pass many of the constraints inhibiting progress.

(i) South Africa is partly a first world and partly a third world country. The driving commitment of the nursing profession to meet the most pressing health care needs and to prepare nurses to feed the hungry maw of the health care system has sapped the energy of many of those well-qualified nurses who should have been at the forefront in nurse theory development. For a century nurses have been faced with a task so immense that a situation of 'their's not to reason why, their's but to do or die' developed.

A pragmatic point of view inevitably became the dominant characteristic of a profession which has been extended beyond endurable limits.

(ii) There was a lack of well-qualified nurse leaders in the post-World War II years. The leaders held degrees in disciplines other than nursing. The first nurse to obtain a PhD did so only in 1965.

Although university education for nurse educators has existed in this country since 1937, the clamant need for nurse teaching personnel limited this education to one year for persons already registered as nurses.

Education for nurses at degree level has existed in this country only since 1956. The backlog of work to raise the standards of the profession and to promote research in nursing was so great, and the resources to do this were so limited, that very little could be done to work out a theory base for South African nursing and to validate it. All of us had to rely on Florence Nightingale's teaching and on the 'model' provided by Henrietta Stockdale. Many of us defined nursing as we understood it. Some of us wrote books on the nature of its practice, some of us expressed our 'gut feeling' about its enduring principles, and others expounded views on their empirical findings as to what nursing is. But this was not theory building as we envisage it.

Post-graduate nursing education for Master's and Doctoral degrees began in this country in 1967. Looking back to the early years of establishing nursing degrees it is clear that we were debating the same sort of ideas about what nursing is as our colleagues were doing at the same time in the USA. In Philosophical Anthropology seminars under the guidance of the great CK Oberholzer we were debating the viewpoints that Martha Rogers has since publicised. This was a time when we were not as exposed to the literature of our colleagues in the USA as we are now. Subsequently we found that we were saying the same things as they were, and that there was as much diversity in our thinking as in theirs!

However, we did not view ourselves as 'theorists', but merely as seekers after some of the truths of our profession. The reason for this was, and still is, that despite the fact that there is an extensive range of such thinking, the designation 'theory of nursing' was not regarded as appropriate because our concepts were never validated by meticulous research.

The Afrikaans-speaking nurses who were the leaders in this regard in this country have a wealth of material on their shelves which has not been published, but which could have the same meaning for nursing in this country as the work of Orlando, Peplau, Orem, Travelbee, Levine, Rogers and Wiedenbach has for nursing in the USA and further afield. Inadequate professional publication facilities were, and still are, a great drawback in developments of this nature.

(iii) The multiplicity of language groups represented in the South African nursing profession has slowed down the development of nursing as a scientific discipline. Nurses from some 40 different language groups are members of the profession. The majority of nurses use English as their professional language, but for the majority of nurses English is either a second or even a third language. To use a language other than one's own when developing scientific thinking, reading scientific literature, entering into debates and endeavouring to analyse, synthesise and derive concepts from research data is an extremely difficult task. It is one of the greatest constraints on theory testing in countries such as ours. To find intrinsic value overnight in something one is struggling to understand in a language that is not one's own is asking a great deal of any human being.

(iv) The recognition of the need for the development of theories of nursing is a post-World War II phenomenon. Before this period nurse educators tended to subscribe to the concept that nursing had no real claim to an independent existence as a scientific discipline. Both Taylor and Goodrich, noted nurse educators in the USA, subscribed to this view by accepting the concept that nursing had a function dependent on the doctor (Taylor 1934: 476 and Goodrich 1946: 741). Between 1902 and 1944, as a result of the dominating influence of the medical profession and the negativism of the many nurses from the Poor Law Infirmaries of Great Britain who settled in South Africa after the Anglo-Boer War (the South African War 1899-1902), South African nurses also accepted that the nurse's function was dependent on that of the medical practitioner, thereby negating the concept that nursing was a discipline in its own right. Remnants of this tendency or belief still persist, certainly among many doctors, those nurses having a 'handmaiden mentality' and those who are so overwhelmed by the service demands that they cannot spare the time to think about the true meaning and development of the nursing discipline. This attitude inevitably stultifies the development of all aspects of the profession, particularly its intellectual dimensions. It impedes the gains the profession has made since 1944 by boldly accepting a professional code of practice which clearly delineates that the function of the nurse is dependent on the law which authorises her to practice and on other relevant common and statutory laws, and not on the doctor. Her autonomous independent and interdependent functions and her accountability in this regard forms the basis for judgement in a disciplinary case, and sets the discipline of nursing apart from the discipline of medicine although the two complement each other. The literature from overseas, with its emphasis on the function of the nurse being dependent on the doctor, has an undermining effect on the thinking of the less well-informed nurse in this country. In such a situation doubt arises about the validity of nursing as a scientific, independent discipline.

(v) The controversy in certain overseas circles about the relevance of nursing theories, or about their very existence, has also retarded research into the development of a viable and scientifically validated theory for nursing in this country. McGee says:

> We cannot ignore the proliferation of nursing theories. But neither can we ignore the current questioning of whether or not there really is any such thing as a nursing theory as such (McGee 1982: 30).

She quotes Luther Christman's vigorous objection to the concept of a nursing theory, as well as Beckstrand's well-reasoned approach which also opposes the concept. McGee sees this as a healthy approach to the ultimate scientific validation of the claims of nursing theory:

> The negative attitude to the claims of nursing theory seems to us a healthy reaction to the ideologic, dogmatic and non-critical way of selecting and using current nursing conceptions, whether those are called theories or conceptual frameworks (McGee 1982: 33).

There has been a tendency among nurse academics in this country to wait until the dust on these arguments settles a bit. I do not think that this has been a very wise policy.

A time for commitment to action

I want to take a stand today. We have waited long enough to loosen the bonds of our many constraints before committing ourselves to action. We must realise that we will never loosen them all. We must commit ourselves to action now. I believe that we have to harness our intellectual power and do our share of research in this field of nursing endeavour. If the answers we come up with support one or more of the international grand theorists because we have been able to validate their findings, or if we find that theoretical pluralism has more meaning for us than one or other of the single theories, we will have gained immeasurably because we will have been thinking systematically about nursing science and nursing practice. We will have honed our intellects and will emerge as serious scholars in our field. We might even identify and develop a series of theories of nursing with unifying strands, for 'Ex Africa semper aliquid novi' (Out of Africa always something new).

Let our commitment be in line with that of Kerlinger, who states that 'theory development is the basic purpose of science' (Kerlinger 1979: 64).

Because the nursing discipline is a scientific one our duty with regard to theory development is clear. The nursing discipline cannot progress unless it is clearly defined, and for this we need a theory or theories for nursing. I agree with Donaldson and Crowley that 'the very survival of the profession may be at risk unless the discipline is defined' (Donaldson and Crowley 1978: 113-120).

To define the discipline there has to be at least a validated theory. 'The development of theory is the most crucial task facing nursing today' (Chinn & Jacobs 1978: 1-11). Let us adopt the standpoint that we need nursing theories as a basis for a systematised approach to practice which will help the individual practitioner to plan nursing action and marshal ideas and knowledge into manageable components for effective implementation. Intellectual activity, before practical activity, requires theory as a tool of thought. Ferrinho says 'the theory provides a comprehensive framework of explanation of the phenomenon to which the theory refers' (Ferinho 1981: x). Van Rooyen puts it even more clearly when he says: 'practice is nothing but the application of theoretical principles' (Van Rooyen 1972: 65).

Menke sees nursing discipline in the evolutionary process of becoming a science. I support this view, not because I do not believe that nursing is already a science, but because I believe that all sciences are in a constant state of flux and flow, in a state of ongoing development. Menke states that nursing can become a science only:

> if nurses develop a highly organised and specialised field of knowledge and concomitantly continue to be seekers of knowledge. The body of knowledge required is theories of nursing (Menke in Chaska 1978: 216).

I would like to modify this statement to indicate that the nursing discipline cannot experience *growth* as a science unless we identify, test and adapt that body of knowledge we now call nursing theory.

My research into the history of nursing and midwifery shows that for six thousand years at least there have been concepts about nursing which some would classify as theories. I am tempted to state that when the division of labour occurred in the life of pre-historic man, there was a definite, empirically tested belief or 'theory' as to *what, where, when, how, who* and *why* certain vocational acts were delineated. Division of labour gave rise to occupational workers and occupational personalities. I believe that the development of an occupational personality does not arise merely from the sociological division of labour into occupations. Workers may arise from this act, but not occupational personalities. An occupational personality arises from socialisation into and close identification with the occupation pursued. This requires that the person understands fully, and accepts, what that occupation in its fullest extent implies, and is able, through the extent of the knowledge base of that occupation, to measure up to persons in related prestigious occupations. It is really a case of 'because I know, I am' (with apologies to Descartes).

In nursing it is essential to know *what* the nursing discipline is. It is essential to know what the phenomenon of nursing is and to understand the underlying theory that develops the systematic thinking essential to the recognition and development of the discipline. It is our task to identify and clarify such theory. In this country we refer to the discipline of nursing as a science. It is science and philosophy which provide validity and meaning to the art. (The Afrikaans translation of nursing science, 'verpleegkunde', expresses this succinctly.) The development of our knowledge baseline requires careful thought about the underlying theory for the discipline.

Johnson, a noted nurse theorist in the USA, points out that all professions have a scientific foundation, a body of tested knowledge that serves as a baseline for practice. She states:

> at the most fundamental level all professions (and that includes the professional outgrowths of the basic sciences) are applied sciences in that theoretical knowledge is developed and used to attain practical results (Johnson 1974: 334).

A body of theoretical knowledge is an essential foundation for the practice of a profession. Without a recognised body of knowledge and without methods for generating further knowledge the claim to professional status is a weak one. In any field of intellectual endeavour theory 'generates knowledge for the improvement of practice by describing, explaining, predicting and controlling phenomena' (Marriner 1986: 3). Therefore we have to look to the development of theory to help develop our analytical skills, to challenge our thinking, to explain our values and to validate our assumptions about what nursing means and does. We have to use the development of theory as the thrust to determine the purpose of our practice and to clarify our thoughts on the social congruence, social significance and social utility of the body of knowledge that forms the baseline of our practice.

I believe that nursing theory should help the arbiters on the academic future of nursing science and the consumers of the output of the nursing discipline to differentiate scientifically between nursing's contribution to the health of the nation and that of other health professions. It should help to bring home to doctors, nurses and health planners that although medicine and nursing complement each other in the concept of total health care, they are nevertheless two parallel and totally separate disciplines, irrespective of how they move up and down on the total health care continuum.

In addition to the generation of a body of knowledge to serve as the baseline for nursing practice, it is an accepted fact that a nursing theory is directed ultimately at ensuring excellence in nursing, for our moral values and the knowledge and skills we define should become more clear when we have a clear understanding of what we are about.

I have long believed, despite the Jeremiahs in the profession, that a profession which does not set ongoing theory development as one of its main goals will become lost in the quicksands of pragmatism, which unfortunately so frequently overshadows the intellectual endeavours of the profession. We have to explore a theory which explains the phenomenon of the nursing discipline in this country. It has to be testable, refutable and alterable.

I believe, too, that we have to make our contribution to the search for a unified grand theory of nursing, to give the discipline a more clearly defined identity and to spell out clearly what its unique contribution to society is, although this should not preclude the development of sub-theories for the various elements of nursing or the various subsystems of the profession. To do this the profession has to 'transform nursing knowledge from a record of unrationalised experiences to a logical organisation of relevant phenomena' (Flaherty in McGee 1982: 140).

A noted theorist, Marian McGee of Ottawa University, has given a definition of the discipline of nursing which, to my mind, is on a par with that given by Florence Nightingale. McGee describes nursing as:

a process of nurse-patient interaction that stems from the assessment of a patient's need and levels of functioning and that is designed to optimise the patients' adaptability through modification and/or reinforcement of the environment, modification and/or reinforcement of behaviour, and biological care and maintenance. The process can be accomplished through the use of nursing care strategies in appropriate measure (Flaherty quoting McGee in McGee 1982: 141).

This definition states precisely what nursing is and what nurses do:

It incorporates the notion that nursing practice focuses on the promotion of optimal health for individuals and families. Health is a manifestation of the competence with which individuals and families function . . . if the aim of nursing is to promote functional competence, nurses in various settings must be well versed in the knowledge, the techniques, and the conceptual and theoretical rationales that underlie nursing practice (Flaherty in McGee 1982: 142).

Extrinsic and intrinsic value of a theory of nursing

What with the jostling of the underground interprofessional power struggles which occur in this country, and the attempts by some authorities to limit the scarce financial resources available at universities predominantly to the older professions and academic disciplines, the development of valid theories of nursing is particularly relevant. The development of an ever-growing body of knowledge is a valuable extrinsic factor in the recognition of the nursing discipline as a valid academic discipline. It is also particularly relevant as an intrinsic factor in nursing's own assessment of its status as a professional academic discipline, for it enables the nursing profession to satisfy itself regarding the validity of its claims to academic stature and excellence. It is also of vital intrinsic importance to the individual professional practitioner, who knows that her knowledge is based on firm scientific foundations.

Are there too many theories of nursing?

I am no theorist, in fact I have an eclectic approach, but I believe that there is a need for one of our intellectual nurse leaders to come up with a unified grand theory of nursing or with proof that a pluralistic approach is essential. There is too great a proliferation of theories. On a recent visit to Britain and Western Europe I became aware that curriculum planners in these countries face the same dilemma that we do. There are too many theories. The approaches of the colleagues with whom I discussed the matter were limited to one of the following:

(i) A theory propounded by one of the better-known theorists is used. I found it difficult to ascertain why a particular theory was utilised; I had the feeling it was something one had to do because it was a world trend.

(ii) An eclectic approach is adopted because no single theory satisfies the diverse dimensions of the nursing discipline.

(iii) The need for a theory is disregarded.

This is obviously also the case in South Africa.

The need to investigate the concept of a decisive pluralism

There is a need to investigate the value of utilising a decisive theoretical pluralism in nursing science. There is extensive evidence that the numerous conceptual frameworks within the nursing discipline could be unified into a pluralistic approach:

> Should a definite effort not be made to analyse and discuss the implications that a position for pluralism might hold in the development of the discipline and preparation for membership in the discipline? (McGee 1982: 4).

If an international conference on this aspect of theory development could be organised, I would advise all the participants in this session to proceed to it with all haste, collar the front seats, and participate in the proceedings with all their faculties at full alert, for I think we might just find the answers we need, particularly if the controversial Patricia James and James Dickoff could be persuaded to present papers on the implications of theoretical pluralism for practice.

Theory development is vision for the future

Let us remember in starting this day's work that the word 'theory' derives from the Greek *theoria*, meaning 'vision'. Last night I spoke about Henrietta Stockdale's vision of nursing in Africa. In a sense this was her theory. Although it was a blend of ideational, idealistic, philosophical and pragmatic thinking, whichever way we view her approach we must remember that theories interrelate concepts in a way that creates a different way of looking at a particular phenomenon (George 1980: 5). This was what Henrietta was doing a hundred years ago. How do we extend her work? I believe that our duty lies in acknowledging that the formulation of nursing theory and the testing and validation thereof is essential to the survival of professional nursing. Without this nursing is not a discipline, but merely the performance of a series of tasks imposed upon nurses by other professions and the bureaucratic system.

To construct a system of nursing, to carry on nursing research, or even to study the nursing discipline intelligently, one needs some systematic method for determining what is relevant to nursing and what has scientific validity. We need theory to furnish principles for the construction and criticism of a valid nursing discipline. The search for a unifying theory of nursing must:

(i) yield criteria for distinguishing scientific knowledge from non-scientific knowledge in the area in which the nursing discipline operates (these are criteria of scientific *quality*)

(ii) yield criteria for distinguishing what is relevant to the nursing discipline from what is not so that the field of nursing science may be defined (these are criteria of *relevance*)

(iii) furnish practical procedural rules for applying these criteria in practical nursing research.

Nursing theory research has a long road to travel to attain these objectives. We need theorists who are experts in the logic of science and specialists in nursing science.

Conclusion

In closing may I add that there is a profound need for the development of a simplified approach to the clarifiction of nursing theories, since the value of a theory lies in its understandability by users. The diversity in the culture, language and professional preparation of practitioners requires simplicity of approach if important theories are to obtain national or even international acceptance from nurse practitioners. Given this requirement, I believe that nurses in this country accept that they have a moral obligation to enhance the stature of their discipline by contributing to substantive theory building.

References

Chaska, NL. 1978. *The nursing profession: a time to speak*. New York: McGraw-Hill.
Chinn, PL & Jacobs, MK. 1978. A model for theory development in nursing. *Journal of Advanced Nursing Science*, 1(1): 1-11.
Donaldson, SK & Crowley, DM. 1978. The discipline of Nursing. *Nursing Outlook*, 26: 113-120.
Ferinho, H. 1981. *Towards a theory of community social work*. Cape Town: Juta.
George, JB. 1980. *Nursing theories. The base for professional nursing practice*. 2nd ed. Englewood Cliffs, NJ.: Prentice Hall Inc.
Goodrich, A. 1946. A definition of nursing. *American Journal of Nursing*, 46: 741.
Johnson, DE. 1974. Development of theory: A requisite for nursing as a primary health profession. *Nursing Research*, 15(5): 372-377.
Kerlinger, F. 1979. *Behavioral research. A conceptual approach*. New York: Holt, Rinehart and Winston.
Marriner, A. 1986. *Nursing theorists and their work*. St Louis: CV Mosby Co.
McGee, M. 1982. *Theoretical pluralism in nursing science*. Ottawa University: Ottawa Press.
Nightingale, F. 1859. *Notes on Nursing. What it is and what it is not*. Harrison reprint 1980. London: Churchill Livingstone.
Taylor, E. 1934. What is the nature of nursing? *American Journal of Nursing*, 34: 476.
Van Rooyen, IJJ. 1972. *Report of the National Conference on Welfare Planning*. Pretoria: Government Printer.

Recommended reading

Brown, M. (Ed). 1971. *The social responsibility of the scientist*. New York: The Free Press.
Beckstrand, J. 1978a. The need for a practice theory as indicated by the knowledge used in the conduct of practice. *Research in Nursing and Health*, 1(4): 175-179.
Beckstrand, J. 1978b. The notion of a practice theory and the relationship of scientific and ethical knowledge to practice. *Research in Nursing and Health*, 1(3): 131-136.
Beckstrand, J. 1980. A critique of several conceptions of practice theory in nursing. *Research in Nursing and Health*, 3: 69-79.
Christman, L. 1977. Moral dilemmas for practitioners in a changing society. *Journal of Nursing Administration*, 3: 15-17.
Ellis, R. 1968. Characteristics of significant theories. *Nursing Research*, 17: 217-222.
Fawcett, J. 1978. The relationship between theory and research − a double helix. *Advanced Nursing Science*, 1: 58.
Fawcett, J. 1984. *Analysis and evaluation of conceptual models of nursing*. Philadelphia: FA Davis and Co.
Flaskerud, JH & Halloran, E. 1980. Areas of agreement in nursing theory development. *Advanced Nursing Science*, 3(1): 1-7.
George, JB. 1985. *Nursing theories: The base for professional nursing practice*. 2nd ed. Englewood Cliffs, NJ: Prentice Hall Inc.
Gudmundsen, AM. 1979. The conduct of inquiry into nursing, *Nursing Forum*, 18: 52-59.
Jacox, A. 1974. Theory construction in nursing − an overview. *Nursing Research*, 23: 4-13.
Johnson, D. 1959. The nature of nursing science. *American Journal of Nursing*, 59: 291-294.
Johnson, D. 1968. Theory of nursing borrowed and unique. *Nursing Research*, 17: 206-209.
King, I. 1978. The 'why' of theory development. In *Theory development: What, why, how?*. Publication No 15-1708. New York: National League for Nursing.

King, I. 1981. *A theory of nursing systems, concepts and process.* New York: John Wiley and Sons.

Machione, J. 1985. Evolution of theories for nursing. In De Young, L. *Dynamics of Nursing.* 5th ed. St Louis: CV Mosby Co.

Newman, M. 1979. *Theory development in nursing.* Philadelphia: FA Davis and Co.

Orem, DE. 1971. *Nursing: Concepts of practice.* New York: McGraw-Hill.

Orlando, I. 1961. *The dynamic nurse-patient relationship.* New York: GP Putnam's Sons.

Parse, R. 1981. *Man-living-health: a theory of nursing.* New York: John Wiley and Sons.

Patterson, J. 1978. The tortuous way toward nursing theory. In *Theory development: What, why and how?* Publication No 15-1708. New York: National League for Nursing.

Peplau, H. 1962. *Interpersonal relations in nursing.* New York: GP Putnam's Sons.

Rinehart, J. 1978. The 'how' of theory development in nursing. In *Theory development: What, why, how?* Publication No 15-1708. New York: National League for Nursing.

Rogers, M. 1970. *An introduction to the theoretical basis of nursing.* Philadelphia: FA Davis and Co.

Stevens, B. 1979. *Nursing theory – analysis, application and evaluation.* Boston: Little Brown.

Walker, LO & Avant, KC. 1983. *Strategies for theory construction in nursing.* Norwalk, Connecticut: Appelton-Century-Crofts.

Wiedenbach, E. 1964. *On nursing. A helping art.* New York: Springer Publishing Co.

A philosophical perspective

16

Henrietta Stockdale Memorial Lecture:
Nursing is the concern of all citizens

[A 1984 perspective]

Introductory commentary

It is the duty of the nursing profession to bring home to the public that it should have a special concern for the profession, which provides one of the indispensable human services such as teaching. It is also necessary that the profession should know how to highlight the contributions of its founders to the general development of the country, and the nature and extent of the nursing service it provides.

Such a presentation presents aspects of the ethos of nursing which are not generally apparent to the general public.

THE ADDRESS

Introduction

Today we remember, and give thanks for, the work of Sister Henrietta Stockdale of the Anglican Sisterhood of St Michael and All Angels.

Her work has meaning for all the members of all the health professions in Southern Africa, and indeed for all citizens of the countries in this region. What is this priceless heritage bequeathed to us by Henrietta Stockdale? Why is it necessary to speak to prominent citizens about it? Do we as citizens of this part of Africa have an obligation now and in the future to think about the role played by Henrietta Stockdale in laying the foundations of professional nursing in South Africa, and in the development of health services in this country?

Sister Henrietta Stockdale of the Order of St Michael and All Angels

Henrietta Stockdale, the daughter of an Anglican clergyman of Nottinghamshire, England, grew up in a cultured atmosphere enriched by a deep awareness of one's duty to the church, the cause of its missions and the alleviation of suffering. She came to South Africa in 1874 as an associate of the Bloemfontein Mission of the Anglican Church. She came to serve in the fields of education and nursing. For this purpose she had received a classical education from her father and had undergone some training as a nurse. In June 1877 she professed as a Sister of the Order of St Michael and All Angels in Bloemfontein. She was the first person in South Africa to profess as a religious sister, and did so in the first order to be established as a purely South African one.

Sister Henrietta arrived in South Africa during a difficult period in its history. The economy of the country was a pastoral one, but the discovery of diamonds led to political intrigue and an influx of fortune seekers from all over the world. This led to considerable social disorganisation and a need for health care facilities. In addition, the almost total lack of education facilities for women north of the Orange River, as well as the lack of organised health services and the need for mission work among the non-white people of the area, created an urgent demand for women of high intellect, imbued with moral courage, compassion, initiative and great determination, to do something about the education of women and the nursing of the sick. This work was undertaken by the Order.

The desperate need for health care on the diamond fields of Kimberley started Sister Henrietta on her life's work in nursing and in the development of health care facilities.

Her legacy

It was the concern of prominent businessmen and leading doctors about the almost total lack of health facilities and nursing care on the diggings that brought Sister Henrietta and her co-workers to Kimberley.

A rare partnership developed between this remarkable woman and the great business, political, medical and religious leaders of the day. Henrietta realised, and made no hesitation in proclaiming in forceful terms, that health care was the cornerstone of economic progress. It was not only a charitable service, but a service which would lead to economic development. She managed to convince the community leaders that developments in health care would not be possible if they did not commit themselves to the ideal of the community's duty with regard to the provision of health care facilities and its obligation to support the nursing profession in carrying out its allotted task. Cecil Rhodes, Dr Jamieson, Governors Southey and Lock, Dr Guybon Atherstone, Dr Arnold Hirst Watkins and all the leading doctors of the day in the Cape Colony, as well as members of the Legislative Assembly on both sides of the House, became her staunch supporters. This indicates her gifts as an innovator and an organiser.

The diplomacy with which she won over the leaders of the land and their unstinting support for the work she did give us our heritage. She could not have done it alone – the challenges were too great for one person to meet. If the community leaders had not been convinced of the importance of the causes she espoused, they would not have supported her.

The splendid vision of a dedicated nurse and the unstinting support of wise medical practitioners and community leaders who understood the problems and were themselves committed to the development of the country and its health services gave the South African nursing profession a priceless heritage and made South Africa a world leader in some aspects of nursing as early as 1891. This legacy will be discussed in terms of four important aspects of the development of nursing in South Africa.

Statutory recognition of the nursing profession

In 1891 the Colony of the Cape of Good Hope became the first country in the world to register nurses and midwives as professional practitioners.

International professional registration is now considered to be the 'hallmark' of the practitioner in a health profession. Such registration is known as state registration, and with it came such additional world 'firsts' as:

(i) the statutory recognition of nursing schools
(ii) a legally recognised system of education and training for nurses
(iii) national examination and certification of nurses
(iv) statutory provision for disciplinary control of the nursing profession
(v) the entrenchment of the concept of professional accountability.

Nursing education based on the needs of the country

The system of nursing education and training introduced by Sister Henrietta was modelled on the British system. Early on in the course of such training, however, Sister Henrietta recognised the need to adapt the system to the needs of this country. Two concepts which may also be regarded as 'firsts', for to date no evidence has been uncovered that such concepts existed anywhere else in the world at that time, emerged from this pragmatic approach to education. These were the following:

(i) It is not only practical with regard to the country's need, but also valid educationally that smaller training schools for nurses should be affiliated (within a well-defined system of education and training) to large schools so as to extend the scope of experience available to the learner. Evidence supporting this approach has only recently come to light, but these days it is a well-entrenched concept which enables even small communities to participate in the education of nurses.

(ii) Nursing education should be part of the system of advanced education of the country, enjoying the same status as teacher training and receiving its support from the financial resources of the state. At that time no other nurse leader in the world appeared to be thinking along these lines and this approach was adopted only much later in other countries.

The nurses of South Africa recognised the importance of these concepts and for close on a century struggled towards their practical realisation. World wars, economic depressions and the interference of bureaucracy delayed their implementation. It is with pride and a deep sense of gratitude that we may now report that the ideal has been realised.

A philosophy of service

One of the most cherished aspects of the heritage bequeathed by Sister Henrietta is the deep and abiding philosophy of nursing that enriches the professional life of the nurse and is the supreme gift that the nurses of this country bring to all its people, irrespective of race, colour, creed or socio-economic status. This philosophy has its roots in the following beliefs:

(i) Nurses are nation builders concerned with the health needs of every citizen from before birth to death at an advanced age.

(ii) The nursing profession and the community must work closely together in the health care situation to achieve the best results.

(iii) The nursing and medical professions must support each other loyally at all times to achieve the well-being of those they jointly serve.

(iv) Nurses must be committed to the well-being of society and must practise their profession within the parameters of the high ethical values subscribed to by the foundress of professional nursing in South Africa.

(v) Trustworthiness, competence and self-reliance, as well as co-operation with the medical profession and with community leaders, are essential ingredients for success.

(vi) The strength and the progress of the profession flow from the professional association and its commitment to the welfare of the nurse which at the same time always considers the well-being of the community served by the nursing profession. It is for this reason, as well as for ethical reasons, that the nursing profession has outlawed strikes as a means of achieving its particular aims. The profession cannot countenance a situation where the patient is used as a bargaining counter for obtaining social and economic improvements. Nurses in South Africa have proved time and again that they can achieve more by behaving as true professionals and stating their case with courage, determination, reason, responsibility and dignity.

(vii) Every human life has worth and is entitled to the best care that the nurse is able to give, with due regard for her personal beliefs, dignity and needs. This was the essence of the nursing beliefs and the nursing care provided by Henrietta Stockdale, and is still the essence of nursing care in South Africa. It is the essence of the care to which each member of this audience is entitled.

The principle of accountability

Registration as a professional nurse incorporates the principle of accountability, but the philosophy of nursing in South Africa has taken this principle beyond what is laid down by the law governing registration. The principle of accountability has become the kingpin of professionalism in nursing. Accountability to the public and to one's peers lies at its core. We pride ourselves on the fact that the majority of nurses in this country are deeply aware of the significance of this concept.

The growth of the profession in South Africa

At the beginning of the 20th century there were less than 100 professional nurses in the two colonies and the two republics. This small number had to meet the needs of Rhodesia, Basutoland, Bechuanaland and Swaziland as well. In 1899 there were only about 3 000 hospital beds in the region. At present (1984) the nursing force in the Republic of South Africa totals:

(i) 60 941 registered nurses (White 30 605, Asiatic 1 172, Black 24 142 and Coloured 5 022)

(ii) 19 986 enrolled nurses (White 3 055, Asiatic 473, Black 13 551 and Coloured 2 907)

(iii) 37 571 enrolled nursing assistants (White 8 483, Asiatic 400, Black 21 991 and Coloured 6 697)

(iv) 16 179 student nurses (White 5 571, Asiatic 537, Black 8 164 and Coloured 1 907)

(v) 4 805 pupil nurses (White 1 083, Asiatic 55, Black 2 858 and Coloured 809)

(vi) 4 077 pupil nursing assistants (White 1 428, Asiatic 57, Black 1 868 and Coloured 724).

This represents a nursing force of 143 559 persons, of whom 50 225 are White, 2 694 Asiatic, 72 574 Black and 18 066 Coloured.

During 1983 this nursing force provided the services for some 148 000 hospital beds. It coped with some 4 000 000 patients, representing 14 000 000 patient-days of care. In addition, some 2 000 foreign persons from 55 countries received professional nursing care during that year. Some 300 000 babies were delivered, and nursing assistance was provided for more than 1 400 000 surgical operations.

During this period community health nurses in the local authority services and in the rural services provided an extensive network of preventive and promotive health care, including community psychiatric care, family planning, school health and genetic nursing services. Hundreds of nurses provided occupational health services in industry and commerce and thousands worked in the consulting rooms of doctors. At the same time, an education and training service for some 25 000 student, pupil and pupil assistant nurses was maintained.

Weakened nursing standards will affect the health care system

At present nurses provide an extensive service to the 24 000 000 citizens of this country. If this were to be removed the entire health care system would collapse. The consequences for the community would be disastrous and the livelihood of thousands of other health professionals would be seriously affected. The health care industry at private and at government patient care level, as well as at the health care supplies level, would collapse. These factors alone would lead to widespread unemployment.

The health of the community as a whole would be affected, with large increases in morbidity and mortality. The health of the work force in industry and in commerce would be affected, with an inevitable loss of productivity and a consequent decline in the national health of this country.

Nursing is an indispensable service

Nursing is a service indispensable to a modern society. In South Africa nurses have been so busy with the provision of care for an ever-growing population that they have not had the time to tell the country's leaders just what their contribution to the development of South Africa has been. The time has come to proclaim it loud and clear.

Through two world wars and two local wars, through numerous epidemics, major economic depressions, times of affluence and of unemployment, political strife and shortages of personnel and finance, the nurses of this country have been true to the ideals of Henrietta Stockdale. They have been true to their profession and they have been true to the community. Though some of its members may have weakened and fallen by the wayside, the profession as a whole has fulfilled its role with courage, devotion and dignity. It has never let the people of South Africa down.

The nursing profession contributes widely

The profession shares in policy making concerning the delivery of health care. It has its own statutory controlling bodies, the South African Nursing Council and the South African Nursing Association. It has developed an excellent collegial relationship with other members of the health team, and has enlisted the support of universities to help it prepare its leaders, educators, managers, clinical specialists, community health workers, organisers, researchers and writers, as well as those who may go on to become community leaders in the wider sense. The profession points with pride to the fact that the Mayor of Durban is a well-qualified nurse, and that several nurses have served as mayor in some of the smaller country towns. If the the Aldermen of Greater London can elect a nurse as the Lord Mayor of that region, if a nurse can take a seat in the House of Lords due to meritorious service, if a nurse can be the political head of a service in the Reagan Administration, if Finland can have a nurse as Minister of Health, why are nurses in South Africa so slow in coming forward to take public office?

It appears that the leaders of the profession have been so busy developing the profession to meet the health needs of the community that they have not had time to think about service at other levels. It is time they did so.

Nurses in South Africa have outlawed strike action

It is not generally known that the nurses in this country have outlawed 'strikes' as a means of achieving their own social and economic advancement. Nurses in this country do not believe that it is ethically right to use the lives of their patients as bargaining counters for their own economic or social advancement. There are other ways of attaining these objectives, as the profession has proved.

Community leaders must be kept informed

Every citizen has a stake in the nursing profession. Every community leader, no matter what sphere he operates in, has a duty, a right and a personal need to ensure that the nursing profession goes from strength to strength, that it is equipped to fulfil its role and that it delivers safe, ethical, good quality and compassionate nursing care to all who need it.

To educate a nurse for basic registration is expensive. In South Africa the taxpayer, except in a few isolated instances, foots this bill. All health authorities have to finance in-service education, and many also contribute to the costs of advanced nursing education. It is the right of community leaders to know that this money is well spent and that nurses are adequately prepared for the responsible duties they have to perform. It is the right of the community to expect competent nursing care, but it is also the duty of the community to send its able, morally responsible and motivated young people into nursing. It is also the duty of the community to support the institutions which provide nursing education, not only with its taxes, but also with its goodwill and donations of scholarships for advanced study and research and for the social development of the young nurses who are caught up in a transcultural situation in which they have to adapt rapidly to both the social and technological demands of health care in the Space Age, and the customs, mores and ethics of a profession that has its roots in an age-old Western civilisation.

The triad: doctor-nurse-pharmacist

Doctors, pharmacists and nurses form the core triad in the health care team. The doctor and the nurse are most closely involved with the patient. It is imperative that there is mutual trust and full cooperation between them, at both the face-to-face level and the interprofessional level. The doctor has the right to expect that his closest associate will provide competent and ethical care to the patient.

The nurse has the right to expect the same from the doctor. Both parties must work together closely and supportively to ensure that the patient (who is the patient of the doctor but also of the nurse) receives the quality care to which he is entitled. Members of the public must become aware that while the doctor plays an important role in their health care, he is only one element in that care. His team, particularly the nurse members, contributes greatly to his ultimate success.

The population explosion – the concern of the community

While each citizen has a duty to take a keen interest in nursing because he and his family are bound at some time or other to require quality nursing care, there is another, cogent reason why community leaders should take an interest in the devleopment of nursing, and should do so now!

This country is experiencing an unprecedented population explosion. According to the predictions (conservative) of the Scientific Committee of the President's Council, the population, which at present is estimated at 24 000 000, will reach 42 000 000 a mere 16 years from now. Forty-one per cent of this number will be under the age of 14 years. What this means in terms of jobs, health care, education and development of the social infrastructure, beggars description.

According to the present ratio of health personnel to the total population, by the year 2000 this country will require an additional 9 000 doctors, 3 000 pharmacists and 36 000 nurses. (There is not consensus on these figures.) Of the additional 36 000 nurses it is to be hoped that at least 20 000 will be Black, since the present ratio of Black nurses to the total Black population is most unsatisfactory. At least 70% of Blacks will be living in urban areas, with few job opportunities, overcrowding, inadequate social infrastructures and high fertility rates. A large section of the Black community will be living in marginal socio-economic circumstances.

The community health nurse will be the main provider of preventive and promotive health care and of early treatment of ill-health. Health teams consisting of a minimal number of doctors and an optimal number of other health professionals will be needed to provide both urban and rural health services. Nurse midwives will constitute the majority of the members of such health teams.

In order to meet health needs, and here community leaders have an important role to play, three things must be done urgently:

(i) There must be an immediate increase in the number of Black nurses being trained. Facilities will have to be created for this. Primarily, this means greater financial allocations. The right type of recruits must also be found. The teaching and management personnel necessary must also be produced.

(ii) The community must make a concerted effort to support family planning and to reduce the extraordinarily high fertility rate among the Black community, which stands at 5,2.

(iii) All citizens, and particularly fathers of families, must understand their personal responsibility to maintain their own health and that of their families. This is the essence of 'the human right to health'.

Without community involvement and determined leadership the health services of this country will be in a perilous state and the nursing profession will not be able to cope.

The nursing profession prepares for the task ahead

To meet its commitment to providing a comprehensive health service in South Africa, the South African Nursing Council, supported fully by the Ministers of Health and Education, is phasing out the present system of nursing education and training and placing this function squarely within the system of post-secondary formal education. Autonomous nursing colleges associated with universities will provide a comprehensive system of basic professional education for nurses and midwives and will provide further formal education at higher and advanced levels. Thirteen universities in South Africa will continue to prepare a cadre of nurses at baccalaureate, honours, master's and doctoral level.

The phasing-out process started on 1 January 1984 and must be complete by 31 December 1990. Already five articles of agreement between nursing colleges and universities have been signed. By 1 January 1986 all nursing colleges in South Africa will be associated with universities. At the same time the education and training has been revised and nurses will qualify in all the major disciplines in a period of not less than four years.

At last the vision of Sister Henrietta has been realised and nursing colleges have been placed on the same level as the major teacher training colleges in South Africa. In the De Lange Report on Education nursing colleges are among the four post-secondary academic institutions referred to as having an important role to play in post-secondary formal education (universities, technikons, teacher training colleges and nursing colleges).

The challenge to the nursing profession

The challenge to the nursing profession is a major and multifaceted one:

(i) There is a need to break down the resistance to change among its members and among members of the medical profession.

(ii) The sheer volume of the health care that must be provided to an ever-growing population within a partly third world economy will place a severe strain on the profession's manpower resources.

(iii) The magnitude of the educational and management tasks which will confront the profession in preparing the work force and managing the services, which will range from academic hospitals with multi-million rand budgets and thousands of workers to one-nurse out-posts operating with minimal financial support, will require very capable and skilled nurse managers and nurse educators.

(iv) The drive to get individuals and groups of citizens to participate in the provision of their own health care will have to be endless.

(v) Overcoming the difficulty of making each race group aware that nursing is culture-related and that each ethnic group should produce its quota of nursing recruits will require rare diplomacy.

(vi) The financial stringency of the times will slow down the development of services and the preparation of personnel and will hamstring the work of the profession at every level.

(vii) One of the most challenging tasks facing the profession is that of helping the young neophyte in nursing to become inwardly strong, responsible for herself and her actions, deliberately self-reliant and courageous and to cherish professional competence, integrity and compassion as the key elements in her professional life.

(viii) There is a need to persuade community leaders to ensure that young people who enter nursing will be able to measure up to the great demands that will be made on them and to give support to the socialisation programmes that are aimed at making nurses responsible citizens with a deep sense of commitment to society and to its health services.

Nursing needs the support of community leaders

Community leaders from all spheres of activity supported Sister Henrietta Stockdale in her efforts to develop a South African nursing profession. They helped to give nursing a secure status here and internationally. They enabled nurses to state the case for nursing at the highest centres of power in this country. They gave strength to the embryo profession and gave it the impetus to grow into one that has served South Africa with distinction.

The nursing profession looks to the present generation of leaders in medicine, education, business and civic affairs to give it the moral support it needs and to assist in the preparation of its leaders through scholarships and research grants.

Above all, it calls on the medical profession to continue to give it the loyal support that it has enjoyed for a century, so that together the doctor, the nurse and the community leader may ensure that the health of the people of South Africa is nurtured and tended with competence and compassion, according to the ideals generated on the diamond fields of Kimberley by Henrietta Stockdale of the Order of St Michael and All

Angels, who saw this partnership between doctor, nurse and community as essential to the effective health care of the nation.

References

Booth, JR. 1929. *The care of the sick*. Kimberley: The Diamond Fields Advertiser.
Burrows, EH. 1958. *The history of medicine in South Africa*. Cape Town: Balkema.
Buss, WM. & Buss, V. 1976. *The lure of the stone*. Cape Town: Howard Timmins.
Cohen, L. 1911. *The Reminiscences of Kimberley*. London: Bennett & Co.
Loch, Lady & Stockdale, Miss. 1914. *Sister Henrietta CSM and AA*. London: Longmans, Green & Co.
Mathews, JW. 1887. *Incwadi Yami*. London: Bennett & Co.
Rolleston, Lady Maud. 1901. *Yeoman Service*. London: Letters.
Searle, C. 1967. *The history of the development of nursing in South Africa 1652-1960*. Cape Town: Struik.
1983. *The South African Medical Journal*, 1(1).

Undocumented letters and papers

Verslag van die Wetenskaplike Komitee van die Presidentsraad oor demografiese tendense in Suid-Afrika. Pretoria: Staatsdrukker. PR 1/1983.

17

Sister Emma, Sister Henrietta and
Miss Mary Hirst Watkins

[A tribute from the nurses of South Africa on the occasion of their reinterment in the grounds of the Cathedral of St Cyprian, the Martyr, Kimberley, 25 May 1984]

Introductory commentary

The President of the South African Nursing Association, Professor MC van Huyssteen, asked me to prepare this tribute and deliver it in the Cathedral to commence the reinterment proceedings. She asked me to do it because I trained at Kimberley Hospital, and because I have done extensive research into the life and work of Sister Henrietta and her co-workers. Because I believe so wholeheartedly in the philosophy of nursing propounded by Sister Henrietta, I considered it a great honour to pay my own tribute to these great, but oh so humble, women who have influenced my own professional life so deeply.

Henrietta had been dead some 24 years when I started my training at Kimberley, but for me she was very much alive, for in those days her philosophy permeated the hospital and many of the nurses she had trained were still there.

When Dr Noel Kretzmar, Consultant Surgeon to Kimberley Hospital, said to me in 1934: 'it's your duty and privilege to enhance the work and philosophy of Henrietta Stockdale in nursing in South Africa. See that you do it well . . .', he helped me to understand what it was all about and I willingly joined the band of nurses who believe in Henrietta's life's work. My contribution has been to record her work and philosophy and that of those who supported her great venture. The book I am preparing on her life and work will contain many of the thoughts expressed in this tribute.

We all share in Henrietta's work and philosophy, and this too, is part of our tribute. On 25 May 1984 I spoke for all nurses in South Africa. However, our tribute should be an ongoing one. For this reason I make it available to those of you studying the ethos of your profession, that you may measure the influence of Sister Henrietta, Sister Emma and Mary Hirst Watkins on the development of a South African nursing ethos.

The audience that packed the Cathedral on 25 May 1984 – doctors, nurses, civic dignitaries, members of various professions, the public, the clergy and the sisterhood to which she belonged and members of the Stockdale family – bore living testimony to the indelible impression made on the minds of all concerned about the health of our nation by the work of the founders of nursing in South Africa.

THE ADDRESS

Three handmaidens of the Lord – a tribute from the nurses of South Africa

Our Lord Jesus Christ taught that man's first and greatest duty was to love God, and thereafter to love his neighbour as himself. Our Lord even identified love of one's neighbour with love of God when he said: 'In as much as ye have done unto the least of these my brethren, ye have done it unto me'. With his words 'I was sick and you visited me', he placed an obligation on his followers to care for the sick.

Today we remember with gratitude and bring thanks to God for three great women who carried out our Lord's injunction. The Sisters of the Community of St Michael and All Angels, Bloemfontein, have a special place in the history of the nursing profession in South Africa. They are as much part of the development of nursing as we are.

The ministry of the Anglican Church in the territory north of the Orange River got under way in the latter half of the 19th century. The work of the church was hampered for lack of Christian women to help with education, nursing and mission work. The leaders of the church believed that this need could be met only by a Sisterhood whose members could support one another and who had the devotion, knowledge and ability to tackle the onerous work which cried out to be done. To this end the Bloemfontein Mission Association was established in England in 1863. At the age of 15 Henrietta Stockdale became a member of this association. In 1873 the rules for a proposed 'Mission Sisterhood of St Michael and All Angels' were published in the Bloemfontein Mission Quarterly Paper (BMG July 1873). Only God in his infinite wisdom knows what this action has meant to the people of Southern Africa, and indeed to persons further afield, for this event in fact marks the foundation of professional nursing in South Africa.

Bishop Allan Webb of the Anglican Diocese of Bloemfontein, anxious to establish a Sisterhood that had its roots deep in African soil, negotiated with the Community of St Thomas the Martyr of Osney, Oxford, for the loan of an experienced, mission-minded sister to start a community in Bloemfontein with the help of a few associates of the proposed Order. These four associates had been recruited by Archdeacon Croghan and his wife during their visit to England in the latter part of 1873. The Community of St Thomas the Martyr responded to Bishop Webb's plea for help by arranging for a sister to take charge of the proposed community for a period of five years. Commitment to her work kept this sister in South Africa until her death 13 years later (Edwards & Lewis No date).

Sister Emma (1837-1887)

This sister was Sister Emma, who by then had had some 14 years' experience of community life. She had professed at the age of 23 and served the church for many years as a teacher, nurse and visitor to the poor. When she accepted the challenge of starting a community which would not be a transplant, but one born of the needs of the church in Southern Africa, she was teaching advanced classes at St Anne's High School for Girls, Oxford. She was thus ideally suited to the work at hand.

On 5 March 1874 this humble servant of our Lord, who understood both the need for nursing and the need for the education of women, set sail for South Africa with the four associates. This day is a blessed day in the annals of South African nursing (Loch & Stockdale 1914: 20).

Sister Emma founded the Community of St Michael and All Angels in Bloemfontein and became its first Superior. She carried on the work of the Order from Bloemfontein, but somehow Kimberley's needs made a lasting impression on her. Ill-health forced her to relinquish the post of Superior early in 1887. She retired to the daughter house in Kimberley to enjoy the rest she could never have during her strenuous years as Superior of the Order. Her rest was to be of the eternal kind, for on 30 May 1887, after 27 years in a religious community, she died in Kimberley Hospital (Records of the Community of St Michael and All Angels).

During her period of office education and mission work expanded enormously and firm foundations were laid for the development of professional nursing and of hospital and domiciliary nursing services in South Africa.

Today at this ceremony nurses pay tribute to this remarkable yet very humble woman who, in her position as Mother Superior of the Community of St Michael and All Angels, recognised the innate ability, the razor-sharp intellect, the driving power, the total devotion and determination of Sister Henrietta Stockdale, the young associate who became the first Professed Sister of the Community.

As Mother Superior she enabled Sister Henrietta to unleash her special talents to develop a nursing system which eventually led the field internationally in obtaining professional recognition for nurses. Nursing history in South Africa would be very different if Sister Emma had not recognised the unique ability and vision of Sister Henrietta and enabled her to fulfil her life's work to the glory of God and the benefit of mankind. Let us give thanks to God Almighty for enabling his handmaiden to recognise the ability of those in her charge and for granting her the greatness of spirit to enable Sister Henrietta to follow a path that led to the founding of a great profession. We honour her memory as one of those who enabled the profession of nursing to develop in South Africa. We give thanks for her life of sacrifice. In so doing it is fitting to quote from an obituary in the Bloemfontein Mission Quarterly, No 77, July 1887:

> Giving herself without fuss or sentimentality to the vocation of the Sister's life and taking the consequences of that high and holy call, she came to the Colony, did her work and died amidst the busy din of Kimberley life, and tended in the Hospital by the loving care of those whom she herself had helped to train. It was in short a glad life consecrated to a glad service.
>
> Come labour on
> No time for rest, till glows the
> Western sky,
> While the long shadows o'er our
> pathway lie,
> And a glad sound comes with
> the setting sun –
> Servants well be done!

Mary Hirst Watkins

Mary Hirst Watkins came to Kimberley from England. She had started her training as a lady probationer at Guy's Hospital in 1882, but due to ill-health did not complete her training there. In 1884 she entered the

Kimberley Hospital to complete her training as a nurse. Her leadership abilities were evident throughout her training, for she acted mostly as charge nurse during this period. Upon qualifying as a general nurse in 1887 she applied for membership of the British Nurses' Association, and received the certificate of this Association on 2 May 1890 (Certificate No 1037). The Colonial Medical Council of the Cape of Good Hope recognised this qualification and admitted her to the Register for Trained Nurses on 6 September 1892 (Records of the Colonial Medical Council).

Sister Henrietta promptly assigned her to district midwifery duties, during the course of which she received her training as a midwife under the guidance of local doctors and Sister Henrietta and Sister Catherine Booth. She sat for the Colonial Medical Council's midwifery examination in Port Elizabeth on 30 June 1893 and was registered as a midwife on 7 July 1893 (Records of the Colonial Medical Council).

When notification of her registration reached her in Kimberley, Sister Henrietta asked her to take on the local training of midwives. She promised to give Sister Henrietta her answer the following day. That evening, after evensong, she told Mrs Mary Cruickshanks that God had shown her what her life's work must be and that with His help she was going to take on the training of midwives (Cruickshanks No date).

She was an inspired teacher of midwifery. She taught that:

> truly successful midwifery can only be done in a happy home, where the father as the head of his household loves and cherishes his family in a God-fearing atmosphere, where each new life is welcomed as the gift of the Creator, and where the mother of the household is happy to bring new life into the world, and will serve her husband and family with devotion and loyalty. Where these things are lacking the midwife needs to specially entreat the Holy Father to give her wisdom to deal with the problems she will inevitably find there (notes by the late Miss J Tyre: 'The development of midwifery training in South Africa').

Miss Watkins was South Africa's first nurse midwifery teacher, honoured not only in this country but in England as well. Eight of her students passed the midwifery examination of the Colonial Medical Council of the Cape of Good Hope with 'Honours'. At a time when statutory examinations for nurses and midwives were unknown, this inspired teacher set the pattern for statutory education and examination of midwives and demonstrated that outstanding results could be achieved using poor resources.

When the sisters left the hospital in 1895 she joined Sister Henrietta in setting up another midwifery school and developing a district midwifery service in Kimberley. These became famous throughout South Africa and served as models for other pioneers of midwifery education and services. The ethical code she taught her midwifery students has become part of the great heritage of midwifery nursing in this country. The work started here in Kimberley has made a tremendous impact on mother and child health in Southern Africa, and the high standards demanded of midwifery education and practice characterise midwifery in South Africa to this day.

Sister Henrietta and Mary Hirst Watkins saw sound mother and child care as the spearhead of health services. This concept is as valid today as it was when they taught it in Kimberley in the last decade of the 19th century.

Not only was Mary Hirst Watkins a devoted nurse midwife, she was also a devoted servant of the church in Kimberley. To her, midwifery and the teaching of the tenets of her faith went hand in hand. We give thanks to God for this daughter of the Kimberley Diocese, whose life has been a 'light unto many', and who laid down this life on 20 August 1905.

Henrietta Stockdale (9 July 1847 – 6 October 1911)

From her youth Henrietta Stockdale was deeply aware of her duty to the church and of the role that Christian women could play in education, nursing, social upliftment and the spreading of Christ's message among mankind.

In 1863, when she was little more than 15 years of age, her youthful zeal was fired by Bishop Twells of the Orange River Mission at Bloemfontein and she became an Associate of the Mission. 'From that time, when she was only fifteen, until her death fifty years afterwards, she gave her prayers, her thoughts, her time and finally herself to the Bloemfontein Mission and died in its cause' (Loch and Stockdale 1914: 10).

Henrietta Stockdale's work in Kimberley is so much part of the history of this town, of the history of medicine and nursing in South Africa and indeed of world nursing, that there is no need to dwell on it. Today it is more important to testify to her significant contribution to the development of the nursing profession within the broad South African context.

Although Sister Henrietta was a dedicated member of a religious order, her vision encompassed a horizon wider than the provision of nursing services by members of a religious order. She realised that the greatest contribution that the Anglican Sisterhoods could make to nursing in South Africa lay in preparing secular women of good social standing and high moral values to carry nursing to all parts of the country. She considered it her duty to prepare women of this country to provide competent nursing wherever it was needed, but she had visions that went beyond this eminently praiseworthy concept.

It is well known that she obtained state registration for nurses and midwives in the Cape Colony in 1891, many years before similar legislation was enacted in other countries. Less well-known are the following facts:

(i) She was an ardent supporter of the positive aspects of the international feminist movement, for she believed in the ability and duty of the women of the world to contribute to the social and moral development of their respective countries and to raise the status of women in society (Records of the ICN, the ICW and Mrs Bedford Fenwick).

(ii) She believed in the unifying and developmental power of a professional association (Records of the BNA).

(iii) Through state registration of nurses, South Africa became the first country in the world to recognise nursing education legally, approve nursing schools, and provide statutory curricula and examinations for nurses.

(iv) Legislation empowering state registration for nurses and midwives established nursing as a profession on a par with medicine rather than as an adjunct to the medical profession, although it took nurses many years to realise this.

For Henrietta these achievements were but the beginning. She recognised the need to obtain from the Superintendent-General of Education formal recognition of nursing education as part of the educational system of the country, on a par with teacher training which is financed from public funds. In addition to the report of the Cape Medical Committee, which mentions this concept in 1890, her letters to the Superintendent-General of Education of the Colony of the Cape of Good Hope bear eloquent testimony to her drive to get nursing education recognised as part of the educational system of the country.

It is indeed a fitting tribute to the memory of this great pioneer nurse that in the year of the reinterment of her mortal remains, 73 years after her death, the first nursing colleges associated with universities have come into existence. They are financed from public funds and approved by the Minister of Education as post-secondary educational institutions in association with universities, with articles of agreement and a status within the university ambit on a par with that of teacher training colleges.

God moves in mysterious ways to acknowledge the work of his true servants. Quite accidentally, through a series of unforeseen circumstances, a key person on the Council of the Henrietta Stockdale Nursing College decided a fortnight ago that he could attend the inaugural meeting of this Council only if it was held on the morning of 25 May 1984. The result was that the college which bears Henrietta's name formally inaugurated its legally constituted College Council this morning. At this meeting tribute was paid to the work of Sister Henrietta.

Henrietta's work lives on, but not only in the development of the great profession she founded here on the diamond fields of Kimberley. The moral values she and the other Sisters cherished are enshrined in the ethical code of the profession in South Africa. The spirit of service, sacrifice, faith, hope and charity that epitomised her work lives on in a South African nursing credo and in the lives and deeds of nurses and midwives of all races. On her death Dr Leander Starr-Jameson wrote to the Community:

> Sister Henrietta has done more for South Africa than perhaps any other woman. She has opened a door of usefulness by pointing out to them work which, like all work well done, greatly enriches the world (Records of the CSM & AA).

Sister Henrietta had the rare gift of persuading the mighty of the land to espouse her cause. Governors, prime ministers, politicians, leaders in industry and commerce, leaders in the church and the medical profession, and the leading women in society supported her work.

Bishop Gaul, who knew her all the time she was in Africa, summed up her life of service when he said that he 'thanks God for all the inspiration that flowed forth continuously from a life dedicated and a heart and will consecrated perseveringly and zealously to the service of God and man' (Loch and Stockdale 1914: 49).

We nurses remember her with love and gratitude for her monumental work on behalf of the sick of this country and for developing nursing into a profession. We quote the immortal words of St Ignacious of Loyala to recall her life of service:

To give and not to count the cost,
To fight and not to heed the wounds,
To toil and not to seek for rest,
To labour and to ask for no reward.

We cherish the splendid vision she had. We have etched it on our own professional philosophy so that we may never lose sight of it as we move towards a new century. We will endeavour to uphold the standards she set and the moral values she bequeathed to us.

Mother Emma, Sister Henrietta Stockdale, Mary Hirst Watkins – three handmaidens of the Lord. What was their gift to South Africa? As they tended the sick, taught the young and cared for those in social need, they handed on the divine art of service in the field of health. They combined scientific principles into an art of personal service, and gave form and meaning to professionalism in nursing in this country. They did it with devotion, rare insight and deep humility. This also is part of their gift to us. If you seek their monument – look around you. Look at the great health services in this country, the role of nurse administrators, nurse educators, nurses at the bedside and nurses in the community. Look at the great professional association, the educational programmes for nurses, and at the South African Nursing Council, which today directs professional nursing standards in South Africa. Above all, look at the millions of South Africans who need the care of nurses and will receive it because Sister Emma, Sister Henrietta and Mary Hirst Watkins came to Kimberley as handmaidens of the Lord, for the blessing of mankind on this subcontinent.

References and select bibliography

Booth, JR. 1929. *The care of the sick – Yesterday and today*. Historical sketch of the Kimberley Hospital. Kimberley: The DFA Printer.

Bloemfontein Mission Quarterly, July 1873, No 77 1887.

Cruickshanks, M. No date. *Nursing in Kimberley at the turn of the century*. (Notes in possession of the late Mrs AS Bennett, 1 Warren Street, Kimberley.)

Edwards, C & Lewis, C. No date. *Historical records of the Church of the Province of South Africa*. London: SPCK.

Loch, Lady & Stockdale, Miss. 1914. *Sister Henrietta CSM & AA*. Bloemfontein, Kimberley 1874-1911. London: Longmans, Green & Co.

Matthews, JW. 1887. *Incwadi Yami*. London: Sampson Low.

Records of the Community of St Michael and All Angels. Bloemfontein.

Records of the Royal British Nurses' Association. London.

Registers and records fo the Colonial Medical Council of the Cape of Good Hope. 1891-1900.

Rolleston, Lady M. 1902. *Yeoman Service*. London:

Tyre, J. No date. Notes for student midwives on the development of midwifery training in South Africa. (Newington House Midwifery School, Du Toitspan Road, Kimberley, notes in possession of a Mrs Fairbanks, née Lamprechts, who trained as a midwife at this centre.)

18

Truths which endure – faith, greatness of spirit, vision, courage and moral values

[The Henrietta Stockdale Memorial Lecture given at Potchefstroom University for Christian Higher Education, September 1987]

Introductory commentary

When asked to give this address I thought 'Oh dear, there goes the main content of my book on Henrietta Stockdale'. However, my colleagues at PUC needed my assistance and I love to talk about Henrietta, so I accepted the invitation.

As we stand on the threshold of the 21st century and the centenary celebrations of state registration for nurses (1991) draw near, I realise anew what an incredible contribution Sister Henrietta made to our thinking about nursing, its value, and its educational systems

She and her medical co-workers developed a comprehensive system of nursing way ahead of its time. Although its basic conceptual framework derived from the Nightingale System of nursing education, Henrietta's system was based on the needs of this country. It had its flaws and inconsistencies, but it also had two great strengths – it was designed to meet the needs of the people of Southern Africa and all concerned with health care had faith in it.

The enduring truths inherent in Henrietta's work live on. A century ago she set our feet on a particular path. We are still following that path, trying to fulfil our chosen destiny. As we move along it, the beacons she lit still guide the way for us.

THE ADDRESS

Introduction

Today we meet to honour the memory of Sister Henrietta Stockdale of the Anglican Community of St Michael and All Angels. When recalling the great contribution of Sister Henrietta Stockdale to the development of nursing in Southern Africa on previous occasions we looked at the contributions she made to the development of a health care system for this country, the nursing education system she established, the system of state registration for nurses and midwives which came into existence as a result of her labours, the extent of the services she rendered, and the meaning of her life's work for this country. We also looked at her as the leading career woman of her time in South Africa, as a member of the world's first feminist movement, and as a leader in international nursing affairs.

So we have looked at Sister Henrietta's accomplishments, but this is not enough. We must also look inwards, and tonight it is necessary to look at some of the enduring truths, such as faith, greatness of spirit, vision, courage and moral values, that permeated Henrietta's work. These truths lie enshrined in certain events which occurred a century ago. Through her courage and vision, her faith in what she was doing and in the Divine help she could draw upon, the moral values she espoused, the greatness of spirit of her Superior in the Community of St Michael and All Angels and the loyal support of her co-workers, these truths have become interwoven in our history. Indeed, they are part of the very fabric of the nursing profession in this country, even if the fabric wears thin at times and becomes frayed at the edges.

It is an opportune time and place to examine certain events which took place exactly a hundred years ago and to relate them to the development of nursing during the century that has just elapsed and to the theme of this memorial lecture. At the same time we should ask ourselves whether these events have renewed meaning for the nursing profession in the troublesome times in which we live.

I have selected five events of 1887 which, singly and collectively, have exerted great influence on the development of nursing and our nursing philosophy and, if given their rightful place in our history, will continue to do so because they contain the truths which are the cement of our profession, which bind us and our various activities into a unified whole.

The opening of the chapel at Kimberley, 29 September 1887 (Buss & Vincent 1976: 94)

This chapel, which is part of our precious heritage, is now a National Monument under the auspices of the National Monuments Commission. Henrietta erected the chapel to provide the sisters and nurses at the Kimberley Nursing School with a spiritual sanctuary. She believed that nurses as a group had great potential to uplift the people of the Dark Continent if they carried out their role within the scope of a religious faith. Henrietta wanted the chapel to be a symbol to all nurses that Western nursing was deeply rooted in the Christian faith and for this reason, although she was an Anglican religious sister, she ensured that the chapel was always available to all Christian denominations.

Nurses on the diamond fields found it difficult to cope with the incredible political tensions, the social problems, stresses and conflicts which made caring for the health of the emerging pluralistic society so difficult. Their religious faith and the calm and solace they found in the chapel helped the pioneer nurses to fulfil their great task. One hundred years later we have to ask whether there is not a deep and urgent need for the nursing profession in this country to renew its strength through religious faith and actions. This is a question each one of us must ask ourselves. In our highly pluralistic society nurses are bridge builders, and we have often proved that the one great common denominator among the majority of the people of our country is our reverence for each other's religious views. In common worship we have healed many scars. I believe the centenary of the nurses' chapel at Kimberley has meaning for all nurses. Like Henrietta we must ask the question anew: 'From whence cometh my strength?'

A centenary memorial service is being held in the chapel on Sunday 27 September 1987. Special prayers for our profession and for our country will be offered during this service.

Death of Mother Emma, 30 May 1887 (Searle 1984: 2)

It was only after the death of Mother Emma, Superior of the Order of the Community of St Michael and all Angels, that the extent of this humble woman's contribution to the development of the work of the Anglican Church in South Africa, and in particular to the development of nursing as a profession in this region, was recognised.

Mother Emma had the greatness of spirit and the insight to recognise 'the innate ability, the razor-sharp intellect, the driving power, the total devotion and determination' of one of her subordinates, Sister Henrietta Stockdale, the first professed sister of the Order. Quite contrary to usual practice in community life, she enabled Henrietta 'to unleash her special talents to develop a nursing system which eventually led the field internationally in obtaining professional recognition for nurses. Nursing history in South Africa would be very different if Mother Emma had not recognised the unique ability of Sister Henrietta and enabled her to fulfil her life's work.'

It is this greatness of spirit to which I draw your attention tonight. Never in our history has there been so great a need for nurse leaders to manifest the 'greatness of spirit' that will set our younger leaders free to tackle the problems of our times with new vision and in new ways. We cannot resolve the problems of our times with pre-World War II methods. Our problems are too complex and our social system and human attitudes have changed too greatly since those times. Our young nurses are trying new ways of solving our new problems. They are no less concerned than we are. Never for a moment believe that they do not share our concern. Our greatness of spirit, like that of Mother Emma, must sustain those who are blazing new trails. With our wisdom, knowledge and experience we must back them up, uphold them if they stumble along the way. Never for a moment should we forget that *they* are our tomorrow. Mother Emma's gift to nursing in this country is beyond price. Henrietta was the first to acknowledge that Mother Emma set her free to do her life's work.

Mary Hirst Watkins qualifies as a nurse, Kimberley 1887 (Searle 1984: 5 and Buss & Vincent 1976: 95)

Another event that had far-reaching effects on nursing education, and on midwifery in particular, in South Africa was the qualification of Mary Hirst Watkins as a nurse at Kimberley in 1887. After completing part of her training at Guy's Hospital, London, she undertook a third year of training at Kimberley to equip her for nursing in Africa. This year of professional preparation was spent almost entirely doing district work in the homes of the poor. Hence she had unrivalled experience for subsequently introducing midwifery training based entirely on a home care system.

Mary Hirst Watkins became Henrietta's staunch supporter in developing midwifery services and education and in establishing a hostel for working women and a home for unmarried mothers. At the same time she carried out duties for the church reminiscent of those of the deaconnesses of old. Nursing, midwifery and social care went hand in hand, education being the cohesive element. Today we would describe this education as 'comprehensive'.

Mary Hirst Watkins became South Africa's first nurse-midwife tutor. She set a pattern for statutory education and examination of midwives which was recognised throughout the British Empire. She and Henrietta believed implicitly that mother and child care was the foundation of all health services. Her most lasting gifts to the midwives of this country were her ethical code for midwives, her belief in the high standards of midwifery education that are so vitally important in Africa and the foundation she laid in mother and child services (interviews with the MacKenzies, Mrs Cruikshanks and Miss Rex-Wilmore).

Her loyalty to her Superior, her faith in the rightness of her calling and her total devotion to the cause of the underprivileged and the socially outcast enabled her mentor, Sister Henrietta, to expand her work in the health field far beyond the borders of Kimberley.

Today the population explosion in South Africa has given new meaning to the role of midwives, particularly those practising in the rural areas and conducting the midwife-obstetric units in urban areas. Despite competition from doctors for medical aid-funded midwifery cases the majority of babies are delivered by midwives, and with the projected increase in the population this tendency will accelerate.

It is thus an appropriate time to look back to where we started in the morning of our professional development in South Africa. It is necessary to realise that Henrietta chose her helpers carefully, and when she had done so she gave them her loyal and devoted support. By doing this she enabled Mary Hirst Watkins to structure an educational course on recognised medical, educational, scientific and social principles and to bring to it a philosophy of service to mankind and a way to practise that gave form and meaning to professionalism in nursing and midwifery in this country. On the eve of the massive expansion of nursing and midwifery education that must take place if we are to provide the health services that are necessary, it is imperative to emulate Henrietta's example and find a preceptor for the development of midwifery education and services whose work will stand the test of a century of growth and development and, in the process, retain the moral values that gave form and meaning to midwifery education and practice a century ago.

A three-year nursing course is introduced, 1887

Nurse education and training in South Africa had been provided on an informal, ad hoc basis since 1877, and by means of a formal two-year course since 1883, when formal certification replaced the 'testimonial' of the earlier years. A significant change was introduced at the beginning of 1887. A third year was added to the course, which was reorganised to meet the needs of the health care situation in Africa.

At this time a movement was afoot in Britain to establish a professional association of nurses, the British Nurses' Association. The aim was to admit as members only nurses with a three-year course of training.

Sister Henrietta and Dr John Eddie Mackenzie (the first South African-born medical practitioner at Kimberley), wishing to ensure international recognition for nurses who qualified at Kimberley, set about the reorgani-sation of the existing nursing education programme. They introduced a three-year course of training which was regarded as being very much in advance of all nursing education programmes in the British Common-wealth (Burrows 1958: 265; interviews; Henrietta's notes). This course was to lead to the recognition of the profession of nursing by Parliament through the enactment, in 1891, of a law which provided for state regis-tration of nurses and midwives in this country on the same register as doctors and pharmacists. This meant that South African nurses not only obtained the first state registration for nurses, but also became the first nurses *in the world* to write a national qualifying examination (1892).

It is timeous to remember that throughout the century which has elapsed since Sister Henrietta and Dr Mackenzie postulated the concept of recognition beyond our borders, South African nurse educators have furthered their ideal. It is well to remember this, not only because we celebrate the centenary, but because we live in times of momentous change.

There is no doubt whatsoever that nursing education programmes, be they university or nursing college programmes, which do not take into consideration the minimum requirements for registration of at least the EC countries, will not obtain recognition in Britain and Western European countries. Apart from the hardship this will cause the nurses concerned, it will also have political repercussions in our country. Like Henriettas of old we must not only gear our nursing education programmes to meet our own needs, but keep an eye on wider horizons. Our nurses must remain equal with the best in the world.

Most significant about the introduction of the three-year course was that Sister Henrietta and Dr Mackenzie recognised the need for the scope of practice of nursing and midwifery in Africa to be far more extensive than that pertaining in Britain and Western Europe at that time. Care of man before birth, through all the stages of his existence and in all sorts of institutional, domiciliary social, cultural, economic, environmental and disease conditions, characterised the training programme. Preventive and promotive health care relative to the times, psychosocial care and high moral values formed the weft and warp of the educational tapestry (inter-views with all persons listed; Henrietta's lecture notes and Loch & Stock-dale 1914: 49–116). What we now call 'primary health care nursing' was the hallmark of the competence of the Kimberley-qualified nurses who were sent to open up the health services of Southern Africa. Trace the history of these pioneer nurses and you will find that they began what is now known as primary health care, and for a century nurses in this part of the world have been the providers of primary health care services.

These nurses were equipped to cope with all forms of ill-health, with all the diseases then known in the subcontinent, and were taught to diag-nose and treat these conditions in the absence of a doctor as well as to provide fundamental nursing care. In the third year of their course they were also taught how to establish and manage hospitals (including stores, laundry and catering services), home care services and army nursing ser-vices, and how to cope with the social pathology of the times.

Nurses trained in other parts of the empire declared that this was not nursing. It constituted taking on the duties of doctors who, incidentally, at that time numbered only a few score and yet were expected to serve the vast region of the whole of Southern Africa. Henrietta's view that nursing in Africa was different from nursing in Britain and Europe is still valid today, and is still a bone of contention between the theoretically orientated purists in nursing and the pragmatists who see human need and not interprofessional rivalry as the overriding issue.

Henrietta postulated that nursing and medical practice were complementary to each other, and that nursing could not be restricted to the caring and domestic orientated role it had at that time. She and Dr Mackenzie entrenched a diagnostic, treatment, technical and curing role, as well as a caring role, as the fabric of nursing in this country. This was essential, since in many parts of the country nurses and midwives were the only health professionals available. Even in the urban areas doctors could not cope with the work load. At a time when nurses in Britain and Europe were debating whether they should take on such 'medical activities as administering injections, enemas, catherisations and douches, changing dressings, removing stitches and taking temperatures instead of doing the invalid cooking and attending to the domestic chores in the wards or sickrooms, the so-called probationer or learner nurses at Kimberley were being taught how to cope with the health needs of the community and, in the absence of a doctor, to step into the breach and take on the total health care of the patient.

In Southern Africa the majority of nurses believe that Henrietta was right. Nursing in this part of the world has much wider connotations than nursing in countries in which there is a high density of medical practitioners. They consider the concept 'nursing care' to be an all-embracing concept which requires nursing action to move up and down the continuum of health care practice, depending on patient needs and the availability of other health professionals, particularly doctors. WHO has expanded this concept. It consistently proclaims that nurses are the main providers of health care and that nursing has steadily absorbed functions and roles which were once 'medical functions'. Many of the functions which nurses now vehemently defend as nursing functions were essentially medical functions up to the early part of this century. So much for our pious platitudes that we will not denigrate nursing by doing the doctors' work. The role change between doctors and nurses initiated by Sister Henrietta and Dr Mackenzie in the last century has undergone many changes due to changes in health care policy, but has always existed in South African nursing. However, it is now becoming entrenched at an accelerated pace. There is evidence of this countrywide. WHO maintains that more than 50% of health care in the world is now provided by nurses 'who constitute the principal professional staff in health centres and generally the only professional personnel in many subcentres' (WHO 1986: 17).

The problem that Henrietta resolved in her educational programme is rearing its head again. There is opposition in nursing ranks to the four-year comprehensive programme, because too much time is given to developing knowledge and skills for meeting the health need pressures of our time outside the hospital precincts. This is coupled with the objection that nurses are taking on too large a part of the doctor's role, both in institutions and the primary health care services. The answer is very simple. Nurses must either make way for medical assistants or fill the vacuum existing in the provision of health care services in Africa. Has the registered nurse asked what is going to happen to her in Africa if medical assistants are introduced? A patient's stay in hospital is now limited to only a few days and the drive to educate the community to provide its own home care is being more and more successful as health care costs escalate. More and more use is being made of second and third level nurses in the rest of Africa, as in our own region. Our future is in our own hands. How clearly we think will depend on how concerned we are about the health of the people and about the future of our profession. Nursing in Africa is not only caring. The carative dimension is the cement that binds together all the actions, such as diagnosis, treatment, cure and care, that the nurse has to perform because the patient needs health care. Subtle changes in the role of the doctor and the nurse are taking place. We need the vision of Henrietta to enable us to see clearly what our end purpose should be. Our vision or lack thereof will determine the future of nursing in Southern Africa over the next two decades.

Henrietta's nurses cared for patients in tents, in lonely farm houses, in ox-wagons, in huts and in the homes of the wealthy. They were to be found where health needs were pressing. They were doctor, nurse, midwife, social worker and pillars of strength to families and communities. Like the present generation of nurses they had to cope with the health needs of a population comprising many nationalities, races, colours, creeds, cultures and levels of social development. A population explosion and urbanisation in substandard social and economic conditions and the influx of large numbers of immigrants across the national borders characterised the national situation then, just as it does today. Our situation is further complicated by the refugees entering our country from the war-torn areas beyond our borders. Yet, despite the fact that they had to be so versatile, despite the fact that their work overlapped that of doctors to such an extent, they were never labelled 'mini-doctors'. They were highly respected nurses who were seen to be exceptionally competent, concerned and compassionate. No matter what the circumstances they attempted to relieve suffering, prevent regression into ill-health, promote recovery and rehabilitation, and provide such assistance as the dying might need. I believe we have to ask the question anew – what is nursing in Africa? Can it ever be the same as nursing in countries in which there is a high density of medical practitioners, good social and economic conditions and a multitude of other health and community workers?

For more than a quarter of a century I have listened to international and national debates on this issue. Like Kitson of Great Britain (1987: 321-329) I have not found a single meaningful answer that will meet the needs of this country for versatile, committed nurses. I ask myself: Do I want to see nursing by registered nurses made 'expendable', or do I, like Henrietta from whose school I come, believe that the non-expendability of the nurse in Africa arises out of the versatility of her role and her willingness to step in and provide the health care her patient needs, even if she has to fulfil the role of other professionals in the health team? Does not our Parliament see the registered nurse in this role, for has it not repeatedly acknowledged that the nurse is the lynchpin in the provision of health services? I believe this is so.

The teaching of moral values

Henrietta bequeathed a rich heritage of moral values to the nursing and midwifery professions in South Africa. The lodestone of the nurse education philosophy bequeathed to the nursing profession in South Africa by Sister Henrietta was the introduction in 1887 of a formal course in moral values, ethics and etiquette in nursing (interviews with the Mackenzies; Henrietta's lecture notes).

Her teaching on nursing morality has immense relevance to contemporary nursing in this country. Sister Henrietta started from the principle that at the heart of nursing morality lies the healing relationship. Three elements comprise the health relationship – the illness or threatened illness of the recipient of care, the care to be provided by the nurse, and the nurse's profession of her commitment to the patient. These three elements are bound by a trust relationship between patient and nurse, nurse and doctor, nurse and other co-workers and nurse and community. Nursing accountability, which became entrenched in South Africa with state registration in 1891, had its roots in the moral teaching of Sister Henrietta. She viewed nursing as a profession because the meaning of the concept professionalism derives from the Latin word *profiteri*, which means to declare publicly, to profess a certain competence, commitment, concern and philosophy of service. She saw nursing morality, a sense of moral values in nursing, as the basis of nursing actions and ethics. This morality revolves around the actions and interactions of two persons, the one in need of nursing and the other providing for this need.

Sister Henrietta was a leading student of philosophy, ethics and the classics in Kimberley and conducted 'discussion circles' to debate these issues. Consequently it was widely understood by her co-workers, and those whom she trained, that she viewed nursing as a highly moral activity. She saw man as the centre of all nursing endeavour, and nursing education as being 'for the well-being of mankind and the Glory of God'. Although she charged fees for providing nursing services from those who could afford to pay for them, she saw nursing primarily as a service and not a commercial transaction. She saw it as a Christian orientated humanistic service. Love of mankind as an injunction from Christ lay at the heart of the moral values she taught.

It was Sister Henrietta's teaching of moral values in nursing that placed the concept of the *dependent function* of the nurse on the law and the ethics of her profession, and on her sense of moral obligation, and not on the doctor. From this teaching originated the concepts of the independent and interdependent functions of the nurse, which have characterised our professional thinking for a century even though at times foreign influences have threatened to scuttle our thinking on this issue.

Henrietta emphasised that the nurse should implement her moral obligations to society, but equally that society has a duty to respect the moral values of the nurse.

Henrietta saw each human life as being unique and believed in a source of morality which was the basis for the well-being of unique man as deriving from something transcendental. To her this was the Christian faith. She believed that a nurse needs a philosophy if she is to practise effectively. Central to this philosophy were such concepts as the following:

(i) All men have a relationship with their God, in whichever way He may be worshipped or even rejected. The nurse must respect this relationship.

(ii) Man, irrespective of race, nationality, creed, colour, political status, moral values, occupation, culture, social class, social situation, disease condition or personal achievement, has the right to respect for his humanness. This is the essence of the relationship between nurse and patient and nurse and community.

(iii) Man is a social being who needs the love and support of his family. The interdependence of human beings in all life's activities, and especially in the care-giving-care-receiving situation, is fundamental to the success of nursing practice.

(iv) All men have a need for moral principles, justice, affection and high regard (caritas). The love of one's fellow man and stable moral values should characterise all nursing practice.

(v) Man is entitled to the safety of his person, his property and his name in any situation in his life. He is particularly vulnerable when illness strikes. It is the nurse who must ensure his safety in all these respects.

I ask whether the time has not come for us to re-examine our moral obligations to our profession so that we may meet our moral obligations to our patients and society? Henrietta envisaged that the leaders in the profession should provide guidance to the profession as a whole about its moral obligations as a profession. Are we consciously giving attention to this? We know that patient neglect occurs, that there are untidy, untruthful and incompetent nurses in our ranks. We are aware of the large number of disciplinary cases that the South African Nursing Council deals with annually. We know that many nurses are apathetic towards the Nursing Association and the health care problems of our times. We also know that among us there are nurses who are continuously involved in 'an underground struggle with doctors', which is deleterious for both nurses and doctors, but especially so for patients.

Henrietta's nurses had a truly collegial relationship with the medical practitioners in this country. They were competent and willing to share in professional discussions with the doctors. They saw this as their duty to their patients and as their professional right. Are we not losing out when nurses take a backseat in professional case discussions? Why do today's nurses not 'walk tall' as the Henrietta nurses were required to do? Why do some shrink from the professional limelight and behave as if they are ashamed of being professional nurses?

How do we put this right? I wonder whether the time has not come for us to delay some of the many seminars on this or that speciality in nursing, or to replace the endless debates on curriculum design and objectives of the didactic situation with countrywide seminars on our moral values and obligations in nursing in this part of the world? When all of us have again been made aware of the role our moral values must play in our professional life, our moral obligations will become more clear. We will be able to take stock of the health needs of our country, we will know what role we have to play and what we have to do to ensure that our moral values endure.

A century ago this year, Henrietta and her co-workers identified what nursing and midwifery in the African context should be. Henrietta transmitted to us her vision of nursing and nursing education and her total belief in moral values as the basis for effective nursing. For a century her vision, and the values she cherished, have sustained us as a profession and given us the strength to build a profession second to none. We know that these values must remain our strength in the difficult years ahead. It is we who have to ensure that these values endure, for this is the debt we owe Henrietta Stockdale of Kimberley.

References

Burrows, EH. 1958. *A history of medicine in South Africa up to the nineteenth century.* Cape Town: Balkema.

Buss, WM & Buss, V. 1976. *The lure of the stone. The story of Henrietta Stockdale.* Cape Town: Howard Timmins.

Interviews with Dr Donald Edwin Mackenzie MB ChB (Edin), FRCS (Edin) and Dr David Mackenzie MD, ChB, M Med (Path) UCT on the work of their father, Dr John Eddie Mackenzie of Kimberley.

Interview with Miss Daphne Eunice Rex-Wilmore. 1936. Miss Rex-Wilmore possessed a full set of Henrietta's lecture notes. These belonged to her mother, who trained at Kimberley 1889-1891.

Interview with Mrs Bedford Fenwick. 1946.

Interview with Mrs Davies (née Howell). 1960. Mrs Davies trained under Sister Henrietta Stockdale, 1892-1895, and did her midwifery with Miss Mary Hirst Watkins, 1898.

Interview with Mrs Mary Cruickshanks. 1934. Nursing at Kimberley at the turn of the century. (Formerly Mary Webb, trained at Kimberley 1886-1888.)

Kitzon, AL. 1987. Raising standards of clinical practice – the fundamental issue of effective nursing practice. *Journal of Advanced Nursing*, 12: 321-329.

Loch, Lady & Stockdale, Miss. 1914. *Sister Henrietta 1874-1911*. London: Longmans, Green and Co. (Analysis of some of Sister Henrietta's letters.)

Searle, C. 1984. *A tribute from the nurses of South Africa to Sister Emma, Sister Henrietta and Miss Mary Hirst Watkins*. Pretoria: SA Nursing Association.

Sister Henrietta's Lecture Notes (Books 1–10). Kimberley Nursing School.

WHO. 1986. Regulatory mechanisms for nursing training and practice. Meeting primary health care needs. *Technical Report Series* 738. Geneva: WHO.

19

Issues which affect the future

Introductory commentary

In the course of identifying issues which should be considered in research programmes and presentations of nursing subjects by the Department of Nursing Science, UNISA, personnel become aware of the many issues which present major challenges to the nursing profession in South Africa. These issues also rear their heads in most Western countries, although they present in different ways. They are all issues which erode the profession and the quality of care received by the public.

Only the primary aspect of each problem raised is touched upon here. Their side-effects differ in accordance with the situation in which they arise, and must be identified and analysed in case studies made by nurse leaders and advanced nursing students.

The issues highlighted in this chapter are problems which it is believed could have serious effects on the development of the profession.

Theories and supportive concepts are not dealt with in this approach to the issues and concepts which constitute the real dynamics of current nursing progress. Also, the issues are not raised in order of importance, since in one way or another they are all crucially important. They are dealt with under headings relating to the content of the nursing subjects offered at the University of South Africa. However, there are two issues which are interwoven with all the nursing subjects, for they play a major role in determining whether the dilemmas identified under the subject headings will be resolved scientifically and effectively. These issues are *leadership* and the need for nursing practice at all levels to be *research based*. Leadership is discussed first and research last, for without leadership to start with and research to provide solid foundations for attempted change, the profession will muddle along, ultimately losing its effectiveness as a major provider of health care and as a leading health profession.

THE ADDRESS

Leadership in the nursing profession

Theoretically, all nurses should be leaders at the level at which they function. This chapter concerns leadership of the profession as a whole. Nursing is a social activity and nursing leadership a social process. Preparation for leadership is an essential aspect of professional education and it is imperative that adequate attention is given to it at post-basic level. Post-basic students must be assisted in increasing their leadership potential by being enabled to understand leadership behaviour at the individual, group and community levels. Nursing in this country has been blessed with a succession of dynamic leaders who have transformed it at all levels. Because achievements are subject to the dynamics of the social process, they are never permanent in the sense that improvements and adjustments have to be made constantly in order to meet the demands of the social and professional pressures of our times. Renewal is an ever-present necessity and must be in tune with the contemporary needs and goals of both the profession and society.

The preparation of nurse leaders is an ongoing process. Young leaders have to test their:

(i) own potential

(ii) level of self-discipline

(iii) stamina and staying power

(iv) powers of reasoning

(v) levels of accountability

(vi) performance effectiveness in the work situation, the community, peer group activities and professional associations

(vii) performance at the negotiating table

(viii) ability to stand together with other leaders in the profession to achieve a desired goal.

All of the above require self-knowledge, self-discipline, knowledge of the goals to be achieved and self-assurance. Confidence which rests on knowledge and skill in handling problems is an essential requirement for success.

Nursing leadership in this country currently lacks the broad cooperation with other professional or civic leadership that is so essential for success. There is a measure of divisiveness between the leaders of various segments of the profession. So far political divisiveness has been kept at bay, but strong and highly respected leaders are necessary to achieve this in the interests of the public and the profession as a whole.

Change is with us and all around us. Never before in our history have we been subjected to so many and such profound changes within so short a time. The quality of our leadership must temper the winds of change for the nursing profession and for the public requiring its services. Now is the time for leaders to set an example to the profession – by walking tall and showing their pride in the contribution of nurses to the national well-being and the intellectual achievements of nurses. If it is to be an effective social force, nursing must have dynamic, fearless and knowledgeable leaders.

With such a large percentage of the nursing profession consisting of subprofessional categories – enrolled nurses and the enrolled nursing assistants – wise leadership is crucial to balance professional and public well-being and to cope with the lack of funds and the shortage of registered personnel. This is the most arduous charge facing modern nurse leaders in this country. To be effective they must study many things, but in particular social change in all its dimensions, for this factor above all others will dictate the future of the nursing profession.

Nurse leaders in this country are required to make major and far-reaching decisions about the provision of health care. To do this they must be as well-educated and experienced as other leaders in the health field.

They have to be assertive without being obnoxious. They have to understand complex health care and social problems and the theories and dynamics of such systems, must demonstrate above average competence in the field of management or in a clinical field, and must know how to use information systems, how to present their case over and over again, and how to use power!

Leadership is not management nor administration, but the divine spark that fires both these concepts.

One of the main weaknesses in the production of nurse leaders is the fact that no research has been done in this country (or anywhere else) on the dynamics of nursing leadership. This is a shortcoming which must be rectified.

Apart from cultivating the leadership abilities of potential young leaders, there is a need to prepare such leaders in the following ways:

(i) They should be made *au fait* with leadership behaviour theories and mature students should be given the opportunity to implement some of them so that they may be evaluated within the context of the South African health care situation. Potential leaders must know something about the theories of Chester I Barnard, Rensis Likert, John K Hemphill, Jane S Mouton, Fred E Fiedler and William Reddin, as well as those of other emerging theorists in this field. They also have to learn to identify the theories of South African nurse leaders.

(ii) They must be brought to an understanding of what a vital social process leadership is in any situation. This necessitates that they understand the social system and its subsystems of which they form part, role theory, the interlocking of role and personality, the need to be acutely perceptive, the type and quality of relationships between leaders and followers, the use of authority and power, and the scope of activity permitted or feasible. The qualities necessary for effective leadership and the value of good communication, the development of a trust relationship and empathy must be examined in detail by emerging leaders. How to motivate others, how to identify goals and objectives and how to identify constraints on effective leadership are skills which are crucially important to leaders. Skill in dealing with such situations derives from self-directed learning, as well as from discussions with experts in this field or with other nurse leaders. Assertiveness training, training in utilising nursing politics, and even, to a certain extent, sensitivity training, can contribute markedly to the development of leadership potential.

Leadership is essential for implementing change. The leader must identify the factors leading to change, recognise the implications of change and know how to use strategies and tactics to bring about change, how to support those subject to change, and how to evaluate the results. Above all, decision-making skills are vital. Persons being prepared for leadership must study a wide spectrum of activities in addition to the usual content of either the clinical, educational or administrative field, as the case may be.

How do we prepare leaders?

Today how to prepare effective leaders for nursing is the million dollar question. The consensus of opinion in the Department of Nursing Science is the following:

(i) Leadership training must start during the basic nursing course. The theoretical content of such training should not be offered in lectures, but via group discussions, assignments which will develop leadership potential and involvement of the student in professional affairs and in community activity. Self-directed learning and testing of knowledge and abilities through peer group activities and by representation of the interests of the group is vitally important. This is frequently neglected.

(ii) Leadership training must be continued in the clinical situation, where experiential learning and the acceptance of responsibility are of vital importance and where the registered nurse learns to represent the interests of both patients and personnel. Learning to establish and marshall facts in order to do so is a valuable aspect.

(iii) Involvement with the professional association at a variety of levels leads to an awareness of problem areas and teaches ways of dealing with these. Serving on committees or representing the branch at a symposium or a conference is of inestimable value when the person actually participates in the discussions during and outside the sessions. Seeing that such occurrences are infrequent, it is advisable for the professional association to organise frequent, short activities of this nature to provide opportunities for future young leaders to hone their skills. Many branches of the professional association do this.

(iv) The quality of formal advanced nursing courses at universities or nursing colleges must be of the highest level compatible with the year of study. Too many post-basic nursing courses are not geared to this type of development. A lecture system in which learners are the passive recipients of information still flourishes in this country and the curricula for many courses do not present a future challenge; only the minimum requirements are complied with. Research by both teachers and students into the many variables affecting crucial issues, careful observation in the real-life situation, debates, case studies, workshops, written essays, practical involvement in many of the issues and wide reading are vital. Comparison with the preparation of leaders in other professions is essential. One cannot prepare tomorrow's leaders using the methods and traditions of yesterday. The selection of the concepts having enduring value and the identification of new ones which will inevitably affect tomorrow's leaders are not easy tasks. They require extensive knowledge of nursing in all its dimensions, of the social system in which nursing functions and of the calibre of the persons in the nursing profession. The teachers must be experts who are keen to interpret the social situation and to identify change and new concepts.

All of this will be of little value if the nurse is not willing to accept a leadership role. She must have a positive attitude towards her role and be eager to become involved. In other words, she must have the divine spark of leadership in her.

A competent leader is able to function effectively in any health care system and in any system of nursing organisation. She can cope with system dilemmas and with the ever-increasing complexity of the health care system. She knows how to use power wisely for the good of those who need nursing and those who provide it, and, above all, is able to use collaborative skills in the hierarchical systems of the health care situation. She must be skilled in removing the causes of conflict and in handling conflict.

Because the nursing system is in dynamic interaction with the health care system, the educational system and the social system, and because of rapid changes in the technology used in the health care system, leaders will inevitably have to cope with rapidly changing role relationships in situations which are at times ethically confused. Knowledge and analytical ability is essential to cope with such demands.

Let us examine some of the issues which urgently require attention, or which will create problems if not fully understood, for it is these issues which require wise leadership. Some leaders will be drawn from the ranks of nurse educators, and others from the ranks of nurse administrators, community nurses and clinical nurse practitioners. In some cases a leader in a particular employment or planning situation will have to deal with all these complex issues, irrespective of the speciality in which the problems are generated.

Educational issues as challenges for nurse leaders

There are numerous issues which require attention if nursing is to proceed with confidence to the year 2000 AD. Some of the more pressing issues are presented, but they are by no means all of the problems which beset the nursing education field. Each item dealt with should be researched as an issue on its own, but its spin-offs must also be investigated as and when they manifest themselves in different educational and/or social situations.

The issue of the qualifications of nurse teachers (tutors)

The logic of the system of training of nurse tutors in England must be examined, since this is frequently held up as a model for the trianing of nurse educators in South Africa. In brief, the system in England requires a nurse to obtain either a diploma as a nurse educator or a certificate as a teacher (Certificate in Education granted by the Council for National Academic Awards (CNAA)). The Diploma in Nursing Education offered by the Institute of Advanced Nursing Education, Royal College of Nursing, is a full-time one-year course. The Certificate in Education offered by teacher training colleges is a certificate to teach secondary education pupils. It can be taken full-time over one year or part-time over two years. This certificate course does not include any nursing subjects – the basic training plus three years' post-registration experience must provide this. Basic sciences such as physics, chemistry, microbiology, pathology, anatomy and physiology, sociology and psychology are not taught; the course deals exclusively with educational principles and methods relating to secondary education. A midwife teacher must have five years of clinical experience. She does a one-year full-time teacher's course which culminates in a Certificate in Education or a Post-graduate Certificate in the Education of Adults.

In Scotland the tutor follows the same route, but in addition to the required post-registration experience must also be qualified as a clinical nurse instructor.

Is it feasible that this approach can meet the need for well-prepared nurse educators in South Africa? There are six reasons for rejecting this, and in so doing also rejecting the one-and-a-half-year tutor diploma concept which still exists in South Africa:

(i) Professional nursing education is post-secondary education in South Africa. Nurse educators must be able to tailor, and offer, nursing courses to suit the level of tertiary education, and need preparation to do so.

(ii) Nursing colleges are academic institutions in association with universities. The nurse educator in a college must be as well qualified as her counterpart in a university department of nursing science. She must be able to do research and publish her findings or lose credibility in the associated university.

(iii) The nurse educator must have a deep and wide knowledge of the rationale underlying nursing and nursing education and its components. She cannot research or teach what she does not know, nor can she expect to be accepted by students and her peers if she is not clinically competent.

(iv) The nurse educator must also be educated in the liberal arts if she is to be an effective educator of others. She can acquire such education only through study for a baccalaureate degree or study for a two-year diploma which has the components of a degree followed by an Honours course in the specialised study required of a nurse educator.

(v) The nurse educator must hold a qualification which will open the doors to post-graduate study and research.

(vi) The nurse educator must be as well qualified as other educators who prepare professionals for a professional register.

The time has come to insist that by a certain date all nurse educators (tutors) engaged in teaching in colleges of nursing or in post-basic nursing schools must hold an appropriate degree or degree-cum-diploma or certificate. How is this to be achieved? What will the resistance to this be? What should the approach to the content of such degrees or degrees-cum-diplomas or certificates be? Can the country afford a full-time programme for the training of tutors at this level? How are clinical skills to be maintained and developed? What will the credibility gap be between nurse managers who do not hold degrees or advanced diplomas and nurse educators who do? Is it possible to have all tutors prepared at graduate level by the year 2000 AD?

Changing patterns of nursing education

Teaching/learning approaches in the secondary education system are changing rapidly to a more self-directed system of education. Nursing education must conform, but will it be able to withstand the tensions generated by a hierarchical system which requires unswerving obedience to regulations, rules, traditions and prescribed behavioural sets? The practice situation must facilitate the new approach to learning, while providing the necessary guidance, supervision and organisation which demarcates the parameters within which the teaching/learning must take place.

Changes in the organisational structure of health services

Nursing education must teach a nurse how to carry out primary, team and functional nursing to meet the needs of individual patients, but must also teach her how to keep on providing a health service. Changes in the organisational structure of health services result in uncertainty, loss of confidence, negative approaches and many constraints on human behaviour. What with the undercover conflict between nurse administrators and nurse educators, reconciling the educational needs of students in such an uncertain practice milieu will inevitably create strain on both sides. Wisdom and keeping one's eye on the end purpose of it all, namely patient care, are the watchwords.

The financing of nursing education

To date basic nursing education and practically all post-basic nursing education has been financed by the state at enormous cost – nursing education is exceptionally expensive. As costs rise curbs will be placed on this type of expenditure. Demands for an improved system of financing for nursing education will have to be realistic and the new system will have to be cost effective. Resistance to the high cost of nursing education will become a major issue that the nursing profession will have to face in the next decade.

Formal nursing education beyond the basic registration level

This question has to be viewed from three perspectives, namely those of formal post-registration education culminating in examinations conducted by:

(i) an approved health service authority (applicable only to short courses for listing)

(ii) the South African Nursing Council

(iii) nursing colleges, technikons or universities.

This is an established pattern in South Africa and in Britain in respect of qualifying examinations for the various categories of health professionals. It also applies to a variety of other categories of professional and will probably extend well into the next century.

The South African Nursing Council prescribes the minimum requirements for *admission to the register*, or for *listing* or *registering* an *additional qualification* against the name of a registered person. The educational authority offering the course submits the proposed programme to the Council for approval and certifies that the holder of the qualification has complied with the approved programme and is eligible to apply for registration of the qualification.

Traditionally, courses taken after admission to the register were known as post-basic nursing courses and were recognised as such by the South African Nursing Council. This has now changed. Because the four-year comprehensive course now includes community nursing science, which was previously a post-basic course, a different approach is necessary.

Psychiatric and midwifery courses have always been courses admitting the holder of the qualification to a *basic* register, so their incorporation in a comprehensive course raised no problems. However, there are thousands of nurses who have not completed a course in community nursing science, and this course will have to be provided for those nurses who wish to qualify in this field. It is designated a post-registration course and its content is equivalent to that of the basic course.

However, nurses require specialised training in a variety of fields. The Council has decided that specialised courses to cater for their needs should be known as *post-basic* courses. In other words, they are courses following on registration in the subject which prepare the nurse to provide nursing/midwifery care at a post-basic level. This means that a post-basic course in community nursing science must follow on a post-registration *or* a basic course in community science.

The Council has approved the concept that post-basic nursing courses should all have a common part, A, which encompasses all the subjects that all nurses/midwives practising at a specialised level require. Part B of the programme will be specific to the speciality.

Universities should not have any difficulty in meeting these requirements, since in most instances the content of post-basic nursing degrees incorporates the content of one or other of the post-basic courses.

In future the term 'advanced course' will be reserved for courses at postgraduate level, for example Honours, Master's and doctoral courses. This, too, is a logical approach. The Council stresses that:

> the education and training shall be directed specifically at the development of the nurse on a personal and professional level and that the principles of learning be observed, namely that learning leads to behavioural change in the cognitive, affective and psycho-motor aspects, through active involvement of the student. The development of the ability for analytical, critical, evaluative and creative thinking and the stimulation of independent judgement of scientific data are of the utmost importance (SANC 58/M88).

Further, Council emphasises that 'there is a fundamental need to create an awareness in the registered nurse of the socio-cultural implications of the provision of comprehensive nursing in the South African community' (SANC 58/M88).

'Council considers the stipulation of minimum educational standards for nursing education as the most important requirement to ensure safe effective nursing for the community' (SANC 58/M88).

An important pronouncement by Council is that 'innovation by training authorities and research in these fields are encouraged and supported' and it 'accepts the principle of specialisation to promote standards of nursing education, training and practice' (SANC 58/M88).

A further statement of the utmost importance is the following:

> Council's policy in respect of clinical practice stipulates that the student shall function as a member of the health team with certain responsibilities for patient care from the commencement of their training. This level of functioning shall be in accordance with the stage and terminal objectives of the programme' (SANC 58/M88).

All these decisions by council have far-reaching implications for nursing education in the decade ahead. They will require innovative approaches in the teaching programme, the identification of new types of facilities for practica, and, above all, considerable re-orientation of teaching personnel. In fact, a whole new way of thinking about nursing education will become necessary.

However, South African nurse educators are used to coping with challenges. Their acceptance of the challenges of the times gives to nursing the dynamism which is so characteristic of contemporary nursing.

Other issues

Education for changing practice needs, for changing lifestyles, for disease prevention, for changing health patterns, for changing methods of the provision of health care and for meeting social changes is the dilemma of today and tomorrow.

Other issues requiring careful research and planning are the problems arising from admitting large numbers of students from a non-Western culture into a system of Western professional education and expecting them to accumulate a vast amount of knowledge within a specific period of time while being submitted to the trauma of rapid acculturalisation and professional socialisation and having to cope with the stresses and strains of the post-adolescent period and the need to achieve at all costs, which is a dominant feature of this situation.

There is another urgent requirement: nurses must be equipped during their basic years of professional study to write for publication. This requires language ability and skill in putting thoughts onto paper logically and systematically. Writing is an art which requires lengthy preparation. There is an urgent need for nurses to prepare nursing textbooks for South African conditions and to publish research articles as well as the type of article which informs or helps to form opinions. This aspect of nursing education has been neglected for many years. The nursing profession in South Africa can no longer afford the luxury of relying on overseas literature to the extent that it has done in the past.

Development requires international as well as national inputs. Outmoded approaches to conducting the teaching/learning situation, evaluating competence and designing written as well as oral and practical examinations are very real problems in nursing education. What constitutes a practical examination? The experience of the author says it means many things − it is not only a procedure-based examination. Every post-registration student should add to this list and should be assigned the task of suggesting solutions for a few after she has investigated the facts of the issue. Workshop debates would be of infinite value in helping to clarify thoughts and adding to the ideas about finding solutions to the many problems of nursing education. The testing of ideas is an important component of this type of development of awareness about major problems in the profession.

Practice issues

There are many issues which need to be debated and researched. The following are the most pressing:

(i) Constitutional changes leading to changes in the health care delivery system and in the financing of nursing education.

(ii) Privatisation of health services. While this should present few problems in curative services for persons belonging to medical aid schemes, it does raise problems with regard to the care of the indigent, or the care of conditions requiring lifelong treatment which is beyond the financial means of families and not covered by medical aid schemes. Although the state could subsidise the care of individuals by private doctors, this would result in health care becoming totally cure orientated. Another system for the provision of preventive, promotive and rehabilitative care to the indigent is imperative. Conflict between nurses in private practice with medical practitioners will be inevitable, for both will be competing for scarce rands and cents from patients receiving care from private practitioners.

(iii) The conflict between professional organisation and trade union organisation is a very real one which can be resolved only by the professional association fulfilling its role effectively. (See chapters 19 and 21 of Searle, *Professional Practice*, 1986.)

(iv) The nursing profession must gear itself to cope with modern technology outside the clinical situation, for example computers in management.

(v) The profession must be at the forefront in attempting to change lifestyles which lead to fatal disease or prolonged morbidity.

(vi) The profession must try to prevent nurses from dropping out from the ranks of professional nurses and to reduce the incidence of burnout.

(vii) The pattern of staff development is a very real problem requiring urgent attention. Nurses move about and take up employment in services to which they are not accustomed, or in places with standards which differ substantially from those of their previous place of employment. Nurses are also moved around in the service to fill staffing gaps. Some hospitals with clinic services make the nurses from the hospital rotate through the clinics, not realising that clinic work and family focused preventive health care require ongoing preparation and a high degree of skill and knowledge. This practice is one which leads to low quality care. Nurses from medical wards have to relieve in paediatric wards or midwifery units, both of which require ongoing learning and knowledge of a special type.

Staff development is one of the most misunderstood and consequently neglected areas in the management of personnel in the health services.

(viii) The profession and society place a big question mark over the role of the nursing profession. Nursing arose in response to society's need for health care of a specific type – this is the sheet-anchor of the profession's relationship with society. Nursing has a social contract with society; it has a duty to study society's needs and attitudes and to observe these as part of its commitment to its task. Nurse leaders in this country have stated repeatedly that professional policy must derive from society's needs and involve the community in providing the nursing care society needs. It has to help society to help itself. It must lead society to accept responsibility for its nursing needs and its nursing service. Creativity in predicting needs and responsibility in meeting these needs are imperative. It must ensure that its philosophy, its standards, its actions, its ethical codes and its credibility are suitable to the position of trust in which society has placed it.

Finally, the greatest problem in both education and practice is that of maintaining standards of care in situations characterised by severe shortages of material and human resources and by antagonism to the system!

Research – the foundation of it all

All the issues mentioned in this chapter (and there are many more besides these) require sound research to indicate possible solutions or why the problems exist. Modern nursing management, nursing practice and professional growth and development are not possible without a sound research base.

Research must be a way of life. It must be used to put small as well as large undertakings or activities on a scientific footing. It is the foundation which provides credibility for action. It is not something which must be grafted onto post-registration education, but must permeate the nurse's learning from the start to the end of her course.

Research can be done on a simple yet effective level, or it can be done as a large-scale project. The meaning is the same. It is necessary to establish one's facts before one endeavours to rectify problems, to initiate new ventures and to accumulate a treasure-house of new knowledge.

John Tremble's view

Annexure 16.1 of *Ethos of Nursing and Midwifery* (1987: 197) spells out the essential features of the development of the profession as seen by John Tremble. The beliefs he enunciated are as valid today as they were when they were recorded in 1943. How will future nurse leaders tackle the problems inherent in the implementation of these beliefs? The document is a valuable one for debate and for designing plans of action. Teachers and students have to face this challenge.

The composition of the nursing profession as at 31 December 1987

If one is to understand the challenges ahead it is necessary to understand the composition and qualifications of the profession. On 31 December 1987 there were 125 588 *basic registrations* on the registers of the South African Nursing Council (SANC C2/M88(A)). This figure represented a total of 67 088 *registered persons* (individuals) (SANC C2/M88(B)). The majority of nurses hold more than one basic registration. The percentages of persons holding one, two or three basic registrations is reflected in table 19.1.

Table 19.1 **Basic registrations of professional nurses as at 31 December 1987 (SANC C2/M88(B))**

Basic registrations	Black	%	Coloured	%	Indian	%	White	%	Total
1	5 421	19,4	783	12,9	244	16,5	8 402	26,6	14 850
2	20 260	72,5	4 792	78,9	1 055	71,6	19 873	62,9	45 980
3	2 264	8,1	498	8,2	176	11,9	3 317	10,5	6 255
TOTAL	27 945	100,0	6 073	100,0	1 475	100,0	31 592	100,0	67 085

During 1987 the total number of persons on the register increased by 2 171. This represented an overall increase of 3,3%. The increase in the number of Black nurses was 976 (+ 3,6%), Coloured nurses 336 (+ 5,8%), Indian nurses 89 (+ 6,4%) and White nurses 770 (+ 2,5%). It must be noted that this composition will change steadily as more Black nurses are trained to meet the population explosion among the Black citizens of this country.

There is concern about the slow growth in the number of professional nurses. The economic crisis has curtailed the production of nurses. The demographics of the White population, with its low birth rate, inevitably affect the production of an adequate number of White nurses. It is imperative that persons from all the race groups in this country join the nursing profession. This is necessary not only so that the tremendous transcultural problems in health care may be dealt with, but to add to the rich cultural mix of the nursing profession which has to develop a nursing subculture unique to this part of the world.

When regard is had to the fact that non-White nurses entered the profession in any number only after World War II (1939-1945), the growth in the number of non-White nurses is phenomenal. It is one of the spectacular achievements of the taxpayers of this country, who finance the total cost of basic nursing education, and it is one of the special achievements of health care authorities and the nursing education system. At present Black nurses constitute 41,6%, Coloured nurses 9,1%, Indian nurses 2,2% and White nurses 47,1% of registered professional nurses. With the current population explosion among the Black population, Black registered nurses will be in the majority by the year 2000.

Nurses from other countries register in South Africa

It is interesting to note that during 1987 nurses from 18 countries outside the national borders registered with the South African Nursing Council.

There were 319 such persons, together holding 400 registrations. The majority of these nurses are from the Transkei, Ciskei and Britain (SANC C2/M88(C)).

Output of registered persons from South African universities

In 1987 no less than 338 nurses, together holding 679 registrations, qualified at South African universities (SANC 2/M88(D)).

Nurses allow registrations to lapse

Some nurses still allow their registrations to lapse, knowing full well that it is a criminal offence to practise nursing if not registered or enrolled. A total of 2 913 names were removed from the register in 1987 (SANC C(M88(H)) and 2 838 names were restored (SANC C2/M88(F)).

Males a minority group in the nursing profession

Males constitute a minority group in nursing. There are 2 158 registered male nurses, representing 3,2% of the total nursing force. This low male membership occurs in all the race groups.

Is this a question of males not being interested in professional nursing, or is there a restriction on the numbers taken into training, or is the drop-out rate among male student nurses higher than that among female student nurses? This must be researched, since there are more males among the enrolled categories. The reason cannot be the lack of senior school certificates, because thousands of non-White students now hold this qualification. Is it perhaps because nursing is seen as a female job and the male ego rebels against taking up a female occupation?

The drive for additional qualifications

It is a characteristic of the nursing profession in South Africa that many nurses aspire to obtain additional qualifications in nursing. It is also a feature of the group which holds these qualifications that many nurses do not necessarily use them. Many nurses undertake post-basic nursing courses while they are waiting for permanent jobs. Others take such courses because they have a psychological drive to hold many qualifications. If these qualifications are not used in practice they present problems, because there is no compulsory continuing education for each additional registration. A post-basic qualification remains valid as long as the person who holds it remains on the basic register. Employers have a duty to ensure that their employees are currently competent in the post-basic qualifications they wish to use, and registered nurses have a duty to ensure that they are up to date and thoroughly competent in any nursing speciality.

It is a matter of grave concern that certain critical areas in nursing are undersupplied with specialists in the clinical area. During 1987 only 155 intensive nursing qualifications, 129 operating theatre nursing qualifications, 31 advanced diplomas in midwifery and 127 clinical nursing science, health assessment and care qualifications were registered with the Council (SANC 146/M88). This is a serious matter, for these specialities provide the nursing personnel for highly complex and risk-laden services. The profession will have to give attention to this issue.

It is interesting to note that 31,2% of Black, 32,1% of Coloured, 36,6% of Indian and 36,0% of White registered nurses hold qualifications which they have registered with the South African Nursing Council.

Table 19.2 also reflects that 38,8% of the additional qualifications on the register are held by Black, 8,7% by Coloured, 2,0% by Indian and 50,5% by White registered nurses. Males hold only 2,4% of the additional qualifications. Some of the additional clinical qualifications could provide excellent career advancement opportunities for males, particularly Black males.

Table 19.2 Additional qualifications on the register (SANC C2/M88 (J))

Additional qualifications in nursing	B	C	I	W	Total	Males				
						B	C	I	W	Total
Communicable Disease N	–	–	–	2	2	–	–	–	–	–
Clinical Care, Admin. and Instruction	842	217	26	481	1 566	14	3	3	9	29
						–	–	–	1	1
District N	1	0	0	39	40	–	–	–	2	2
Fever N	2	79	1	177	259	13	2	–	13	28
Intensive N	500	187	42	1 072	1 801	–	–	–	–	–
Mothercraft N	92	45	11	271	419	24	5	1	44	74
Nursing Admin	987	132	40	1 319	2 478	2	–	–	1	3
Ophthalmic N	267	14	9	36	326	25	1	2	20	48
Operating Theatre N	1 055	150	37	1 683	2 925	36	9	4	20	69
Orthopaedic N	431	74	9	324	838	–	–	–	1	1
Paediatric N	721	187	22	614	1 544	–	–	–	–	–
Psych & Neuro N	0	1	0	18	19	39	4	9	47	99
Psych N Inst	61	18	12	89	180	17	5	3	39	64
Tutor	793	158	44	1 261	2 256	–	–	–	–	–
Tuberculosis N	0	0	0	1	1	–	–	–	–	–
Obstet Anal & Resus	51	4	5	333	393	26	7	4	45	82
Community N	2 045	581	164	3 126	5 916	3	–	–	11	14
General N Inst	94	12	0	11	117	–	–	–	–	–
Adv Mid & N Natal N	144	19	17	40	220	–	–	–	2	2
Adv Psych N	–	5	–	18	23	–	–	–	–	–
Oncology N	40	19	2	50	111	2	1	–	12	15
Occup H N	38	18	5	335	396	–	–	–	–	–
Spinal Injury N	3	5	0	10	18	–	–	–	–	–
Adv Paed & N Nat N	10	10	0	15	35	2	–	–	–	2
Clin N, H Ass T & C	542	15	5	13	575	–	–	–	–	–
Geriatric N	4	0	1	13	18	–	–	–	–	–
Rural N	5	1	0	20	26	–	–	–	–	–
Stoma Care N	3	0	0	3	6	–	–	–	–	–
Adv Clinic N	1	0	0	0	1	–	–	–	–	–
Total	8 732	1 951	452	11 374	22 509	203	37	26	267	533

Legend: B = Blacks   C = Coloureds   I = Indians
        W = Whites   N = Nursing science

Student numbers

Growth in student numbers remains slow due to the financial restrictions of the past few years. At present 10,6% of all students, namely 416 Black, 106 Coloured, 7 Indian and 871 White students, are enrolled at universities (1 400), while the grand total of all students enrolled at universities, nursing colleges and hospital nursing schools is 13 254 (6 951 Black, 1 291 Coloured, 446 Indian and 4 566 White). This constitutes a decrease of 1 074 since 1986. This figure represents student nurses and student midwives. The actual number of *student nurses* for 1987 was 10 925. This was made up as follows: 4 264 student nurses were still training for the Council's diploma (the course that is being phased out) and 1 400 students were in training at universities (of these 1 183 were following the comprehensive basic course). The rest were following the curriculum that is being phased out. There were 5 261 students at nursing colleges in association with universities, and these students were following the comprehensive course.

The number of student nurses in training is not sufficient to meet the needs of the nation for an adequate nursing force. Attention has to be given to this matter.

Enrolled student nurse categories form part of the nursing profession

The nursing profession consists of registered nurses, registered midwives, enrolled nurses, enrolled midwives and enrolled nursing assistants. The rapid growth of the enrolled categories is one of the major concerns of the profession, its implications for the profession and for the provision of nursing services being immense. However, despite the misuse that is made of their services in exceeding their scope of practice, in many instances members of the enrolled categories are the only nurses prepared to work in the rural areas. Moreover, as the cost of health services and the salaries of registered nurses rise, it is inevitable that health planners will endeavour to balance the costs of health services by diluting the professional nursing services with the services of the enrolled categories. This occurs all over the world, except in New Zealand, where the greater portion of nursing services is now being provided by registered nurses at a cost which places the concept in serious doubt. Realism is necessary; helpers there must be. It is not necessary for all nursing to be provided by registered persons, but there must be supervision by registered nurses. Research to balance the needs of patients and the interests of the profession is essential. The issue is one that the nursing profession must tackle with the greatest measure of responsibility, with the public good as its priority. It must be remembered that many persons who are on the register as enrolled persons also happen to be registered. Of the 25 425 enrolled nurses and enrolled midwives on the register of the South African Nursing Council, no less than 1 538 are also registered either as nurses or as midwives. This brings the effective number of enrolled nurses, that is the actual subcategory, down to 23 887. The number of enrolled nurses increased by 1 501 in 1987 (+ 6,3%).

Ratio of registered nurses to enrolled categories

In other words, there are 2,8 registered persons to each enrolled nurse. This number would be considerably higher if every enrolled nurse worked under supervision at all times (SANC C12/M88(B)).

If the ratio of registered nurses to all categories of enrolled persons (other than pupil categories) is considered, a serious picture emerges. The total of 67 088 registered nurses must supervise 25 425 enrolled nurses plus 43 599 enrolled nursing assistants. The ratio of registered nurses to enrolled persons (excluding pupil categories) is 67 088: 69 024, that is there is 0,97 registered nurse for every one enrolled person. However, this is complicated still further if the ratio of registered persons to all categories of enrolled persons (69 024 qualified enrolled persons, plus 5 676 pupil nurses, plus 3 824 pupil nursing assistants = 78 524) is computed. This is 0,85 registered nurse to 1 enrolled person, which is a very unhealthy state of affairs.

Majority of enrolled nurses enrolled in only one category

The majority of persons who are enrolled (excluding those who also hold nursing and midwifery registration) are enrolled in only one capacity. There are only five persons who hold qualifications as both enrolled nurses and enrolled midwives (SANC C12/M88(B)). There were 1 347 male enrolled nurses on the roll in 1987, that is 5,3 of the total.

Some enrolled nurses also neglect to maintain their annual enrolment. During 1987 no less than 1 100 names were removed for non-payment of annual fees (SANC C12/M88(C)).

Pupil nurse training

A substantial number of pupil nurses are enrolled for training as enrolled nurses. On 31 December 1987, 2 627 Black, 989 Coloured, 106 Indian and 1 955 White persons were enrolled as pupil nurses (5 676 total). When regard is had to the fact that there are only 10 925 student nurses in training, on a three or four-year course, and that the training of an enrolled nurse is of two years' duration, it is obvious that a serious imbalance between the training of registered and enrolled nurses is taking place. Enrolment of pupil nurse training in 1986 showed a growth of 19,8%. The growth in 1987 was 4,7% (SANC 146/M88).

Moreover, there are not sufficient posts for enrolled nurses (staff nurses) to absorb the newly-qualified enrolled nurses. This leads to two problems. There may be unemployment of enrolled nurses, or they may be appointed to vacant posts for registered nurses. The latter situation is the most dangerous. In such instances enrolled nurses are used beyond their legal scope of practice and ultimately replace registered nurses. The consequences for the public of health care being provided by inadequately qualified persons are very serious. The replacement of registered persons by enrolled nurses raises the question whether registered nurses actually need the extensive education and training now provided for them. With the high cost of training professional nurses, this is a question that the profession must face. This issue constitutes the Achilles' heel of professional nursing. It is significant that the majority of pupil nurses who enrolled for the first time in 1987 hold their senior certificate. (There were 3 065 such persons and of these 2 554 (83,3%) had obtained their senior certificate.) They should have been admitted to professional nurse training, but for various reasons, financial and otherwise, this was not done.

The enrolled nursing assistant

The other category of enrolled person is the enrolled nursing assistant. As at 31 December 1897, 25 346 Black, 8 214 Coloured, 720 Indian and 9 319 White persons were enrolled as nursing assistants (total 43 599) (SANC C17/M88(A)). Black nursing assistants constitute 58,1%, Coloured 18,8%, Indian 1,7% and White 21,4% of the enrolled nursing assistant force. There are only 4 820 males among the 43 599 enrolled nursing assistants (11,1%). Only 472 nursing assistants, or 9,8% of all nursing assistants, are White males, the majority of male nursing assistants being Black (3 754 or 77,9%). Coloured males respresent 11,1% of all nursing assistants, and Indian males only 1,2% (SANC C17/M88(A)).

It appears that the policy among employers is to utilise the services of Black enrolled nursing assistants in preference to training Black males for the professional register. This is an issue requiring research.

No less than 3 159 enrolled nursing assistants were removed from the roll in 1987 for non-payment of their annual fees. Non-payment of annual dues to maintain registration or enrolment lays the person open to criminal charges if he or she practises.

Pupil nursing assistants

On 31 December 1987 there were 3 824 pupil nursing assistants in training (1 782 Blacks, 737 Coloureds, 122 Indians and 1 183 Whites). Of these, 549 (14,4%) were male (190 Blacks, 73 Coloureds and Indians, and 277 Whites). This represents a growth of 9,9% since the previous year.

A masterplan is required for nursing education and training

An overview of the statistics presented in this section would indicate that the development of a master plan for the education and training of the various categories of nurse is necessary. The present haphazard approach which dominates the intake of students and pupils is the result of the individual service needs of each hospital recognised as a training school, and can no longer fulfil this country's requirements for a nursing force capable of meeting the needs of the nation for nursing services in the year 2000. The composition of the nursing profession is one of the two most urgent issues with which the nursing profession has to concern itself. The other is the quality of care provided by the profession. The former is the dominant issue, for the composition, competence and ethical values of the members of the various categories of nurse determine the quality of care that the patient will receive, and quality care is the *raison d'être* for a profession of nursing.

References

SA Nursing Council. 1987. *Statistical returns 1987*. Pretoria: SANC.
Searle, C. 1986. *Professional practice – a South African nursing perspective*. Durban: Butterworths.
Searle, C. 1987. *Ethos of nursing and midwifery – a general perspective*. Durban: Butterworths.

20

Educational objectives make or break the quality of patient care

[Address given at Pretoria University, the pioneer of nursing degrees in South Africa, to commemorate 25 years of nursing education at degree level, 1 July 1981]

Introductory commentary

Degrees in nursing science were instituted at South African universities to improve the quality of nursing care through the provision of in-depth study of the many dimensions of nursing science, which would help to clarify the role of nursing, improve the quality of nursing at the point of patient contact, and produce administrators, educators, writers and researchers to help make quality patient care possible.

It was believed that education at degree level would help the profession to identify its role, functions and goals more clearly and enable it to set itself clear objectives. Above all, it would enable nurse educators to identify the constraints on nursing education and to undertake the research necessary to clarify their aims and objectives. The aim was to produce nurse educators who would feel comfortable in a tertiary education environment, but who would also be able to identify and meet the nursing needs of the country and to understand the learning and professional socialisation needs of the student nurse. The educational objectives had to be sound not only to ensure quality patient care, but also to cater for the development of the profession generally.

However, at the 25th anniversary of the introduction of nursing degrees at South African universities it was still necessary to address nurse educators on such an important topic as the impact of educational objectives on the quality of patient care. The topic was raised because it was doubtful that the nursing education system was resulting in high quality, safe, humane patient care as and when it was needed by patients and in the amounts they required. In the debate following the lecture the following question was asked: 'What influence have role models holding degrees in nursing science had on this aspect of nursing?' All agreed that nursing as a humanistic science had been advanced considerably, but that nurse graduates were still too few in number to make an imput that would revolutionise patient care. The consensus reached was that the objectives were clear, but the means for achieving them inadequate.

By the end of this century it will be necessary to examine the following issues: how clear have our objectives been, how successfully have we implemented them, and what has university education for nurses contributed to the attainment of the primary objective – quality patient care?

Our credibility as nurse educators, as persons who shape the ethos of the nursing profession in South Africa, depends on the quality of the nursing education we provide and on the calibre and philosophy of our nurse educators and the persons we admit to the professional nursing course. We will have to answer these questions: How valid have our objectives been? What impact have role models holding degrees in nursing science had on the profession as a whole and on the service it renders? As the centenary year (1991) of state registration of nurses draws near, these questions must be researched.

THE ADDRESS

A most important criterion for nursing education is that a definite end must be kept in view. This end purpose or terminal outcome is 'quality nursing care'.

Educational objectives in nursing education are the roadsigns which help both teacher and student to chart their way through the mass of social, legal, ethical and scientific material that has to be mastered by the student and her teachers in order to reach their ultimate goal – a professional practitioner who is competent and willing to provide quality care within a total patient care context. The rationale underlying educational objectives, the way in which they are formulated and implemented and the outcomes evaluated, and the philosophy supportive to the whole process will make or break the quality of patient care provided by students and qualified practitioners.

I do not propose to tell you how to identify, formulate, implement and evaluate educational objectives, but would rather ask some questions that we must all ponder over. 'Laat ek met die deur in die huis val!'

How do we determine educational objectives for quality care when the concept 'quality care' has little relevance to the way in which some centres prepare students to provide clinical care? How can there be 'quality care' when the patient is depersonalised by treatment and care provided on an assembly line or 'functional assignment basis' initially designed to cope with a crisis situation during World War II? How can there be quality care when the concept of total patient care is nullified by the functional assignment of students in the clinical care situation and where the emphasis is on things and procedures instead of on the total needs of a patient? How do we set objectives in such a learning situation, and how do we evaluate them? Do we set objectives to meet examination requirements, or to provide competent nurse practitioners who are committed to providing quality care? How do we determine objectives within a nursing care plan when there is no such plan? How do we relate the objectives to outcomes when we derail the process with a functional teaching/learning approach?

The national aims and objectives of nursing education and the philosophy of the South African Nursing Council require nurse education and training to ensure that quality nursing in a preventive, promotive, curative and rehabilitative context is available to man from before birth throughout his life span, within the parameters of societal needs and expectations and the socio-economic and cultural constraints of the South African community.

The national aims and objectives enshrined in the directives for the various curricula of the South African Nursing Council are the minimum standards of nursing education for safe nursing practice in a particular field.

They are the common denominators for the various nursing schools, which are supposed to clothe the skeletons of national curricula and directives with the flesh and blood and sinews of vibrant courses tailored to meet not only national, but also regional and local needs, as well as the needs of the neophytes who enter the nursing education programmes in the particular area.

Objectives rest upon values

The specific educational objectives are expected to be determined within the broad framework of the societal needs, as evinced in the national curricula and directives. This presupposes that they are identified and implemented within the philosophy, ethics, laws and knowledge, skills and attitudes regarded as desirable for quality practice, as well as within the broad needs of society and the individual needs of the patient and the student. If the objectives are 'technically' and 'assembly line' orientated, there cannot be quality care in the true sense of the word.

Objectives are value bound, so if they are to be meaningful they must be formulated within the value system which has evolved over a long span of time out of social, medical, individual and nursing needs and actions. In other words, we have to know what we mean by quality care, what our standards are, why we have these standards, how these can be attained, how the student is educated and trained to meet these standards, and what value judgements have to be made when her competence is evaluated during and on completion of her course. We have to ensure that those concerned with the educational process are true role models for student, patient and society at large.

Davies (1976: 3) stresses that all objectives rest upon an assumption or underlying complex of values. These lie at the heart of the planning process (Davies 1976: 4). Note that it is the values that are central to the issue. 'Values' and 'planning' are crucial elements of the concept that educational objectives make or break the quality of patient care. To translate 'values' into action requires meticulous identification of objectives and careful planning for the implementation of objectives.

Quality patient care – a value concept

Quality patient care reflects a value concept in a particular system of health care in a particular society. Medical, nursing and social philosophy, political ideology, administrative policies and social development create certain social expectations regarding education, economics and technology, and help to determine what is meant by quality care in a specific society. There is no universally accepted definition of 'quality patient care'. However, in South Africa we have certain criteria for determining what is meant by 'quality care'. These criteria are the parameters within which we have to identify and implement objectives.

Criteria for quality care – a South African perspective

The criteria for quality care have emerged out of a vast mix of beliefs and views of committed nurses, doctors, administrators and the public at large. The individual and the society of which he forms part appear to judge quality nursing in terms of a variety of factors. 'The safety of his person, his property and his name looms large.' However, the quality of care goes beyond this legal premise. Safety is paramount, but the individual and society expect nursing to be timeous, ethical, knowledgeable, accurate, skilful, humane, empathic and sympathetic, with due regard for the dignity and individuality of the recipient of such care, irrespective of his or her race, colour, creed and social, cultural, political and economic status. The patient expects care appropriate to his specific needs in circumstances where he is the centre of all activities. He and his needs must form the pivot of the care. Society and the individual patient expect responsibility and accountability from the nurse. Both expect the nurse to provide care within a value system as well as a scientific system. Only individualised, total care provided by persons who understand and respect all the nuances of physical, social and emotional needs in the health care situation as a whole, and of a particular recipient of health care, can meet these demands. They cannot be met by a functional assignment approach, where the nurse is concerned with various aspects of procedure and not with the total spectrum of human needs which bedevils the particular health care situation.

Where are the criteria and objectives for quality care generated?

The educational objectives aimed at providing quality care are generated by and evolve from the same source as the criteria. The objectives have to ensure that the criteria are met. Specific educational objectives can never be divorced from the broad aims and goals of the programme. This is where we frequently go wrong, and this is where a functional approach in our teaching sabotages the basic meaning of nursing as spelt out by Henderson, Orem, Levine, Rogers, King and others, and as manifested in *A South African Nursing Credo*.

Nursing in its true sense, and hence the educational objectives for the teaching of the discipline, presupposes a depth of knowledge about society's health needs, views, cultural values, economic and human resources and political will. It also presupposes a depth of understanding of all the developmental stages of man as a biological and social being, of medical science and technology, of nursing science and philosophy – its aspirations and potential, and of the developmental stages, intellectual potential, philosophy, norms and values and aspirations of the student nurse. In her student years, as well as in her life as a registered nurse practitioner, the nurse has to supply a realistic, holistic interdigitation of a mass of scientific detail from a variety of disciplines in order to provide humane, empathic, sympathetic, individualised, scientific nursing care. Within a framework of nursing philosophy, human needs, scientific nursing knowledge, psychomotor and affective skills, laws, ethics and administrative policies and practices, the mass of basic material has to be transformed into quality patient care.

Clear objectives which take all the foregoing into consideration have to be devised to serve as the landmarks past which the student wends her way through the learning content of the discipline. In a system where teaching and clinical practica are frequently concerned with things in general and not with the variety of human needs which bedevil the particular health care situation, both teacher and student may lose their way, to the detriment of patient care.

Ineffective teaching modalities negate objectives

If our clinical practice system is 'functional assignment dominated', how valid are our objectives for ensuring quality care? It is not only the system of teaching by 'functional assignment' that defeats the identification and implementation of objectives which could ensure quality care; coupled with this is the problem of other teaching approaches which weaken student involvement and the realisation of objectives.

It is a widely-held assumption that presently much of nurse teaching is approached from the 'classical perspective', that is it consists overwhelmingly of lectures within an autocratic, conservative, subject and teacher-dominated, other-directed, over-disciplined, skill-orientated atmosphere, where far too little (or sometimes no) attention is given to factors such as creativity, personal and professional growth, self-fulfilment of the individual student, the nurturing of inquiring minds, participation in the instructional system and the end purpose of it all. This end purpose is not the examination at the end of the course, but the provision of quality health care for man from before birth throughout all the stages of his life. Unless the end purpose, the underlying values, the scientific content and the potential of the student are seen as a whole, and unless form and substance is given to the educational process through careful identification of learning needs, the formulation of explicit objectives, careful definition of the rationale for specific objectives and the meaningful interpretation of objectives, the educational system will at best be mechanistic. How can the student know what path she must follow unless she encounters clear milestones in the form of realistic objectives? How can she progress from the simple to the complex unless the objectives are clearly defined, and how, oh how, can she cope with the reality of clinical nursing if she does not master the objectives at each of the various stages of the curriculum before she is confronted with the reality of providing skilled care to seriously ill patients?

Objectives influenced by how we view nursing education

How do we view nursing education? Is it merely the preparation of certain categories of nursing personnel at basic, post-basic and in-service educational levels, or is it something more?

As a committed nurse teacher I believe:

(i) Nursing education is inescapably a moral undertaking. Those who see no meaning in nursing and nursing education have missed this basic truth. The aim of society in providing education and training for nurses is to supply a service to society. Its purpose is to ensure that a cadre of citizens with specialised knowledge and skills is available to provide competent and humane nursing care within the parameters of the ethical norms of the profession and society's legal, political, economic, social and cultural constraints. These strands, which interpret society's aims, weave throughout the educational programme. They have short-term as well as long-term objectives, which generally extend decades into the future. Every aspect of the learning content has to be seen from this perspective, so all learning objectives must relate to these. This is the cement which binds all the aspects of the course into a meaningful whole.

(ii) Nursing education is not merely the preparation of students to perform tasks in the clinical situation or for future professional practice, it is life itself, for every learning objective should have two ends in view, namely quality care for a human life in need of health care and personal and professional self-realisation and the attainment of 'meaning in life'. For the student, attainment of 'meaning in life' is the most important formative influence of her professional preparation. This will motivate her to provide quality nursing care.

(iii) Nurses are decision makers and problem solvers. Appropriateness of knowledge, skills and attitudes are key issues in the determination of objectives. Receiving their professional preparation in a milieu in which the educational objectives support the societal aims, professional goals and total patient care, and the clear identification of objectives underlies every dimension of the learning process, is part of the preparation they need for decision making and problem solving. Early on in their programme they must learn that identifying objectives is crucial to the utilisation of resources and to all effective nursing action.

(iv) The student nurse has to be socialised into the role of a nurse. The influence of effective role models and active involvement in all the dimensions of nursing education are important and questioning and critical evaluation of the rationale underlying social and nursing care objectives are vital formative influences in this process. Quality care depends not only on knowledge and psychomotor skills, but is inextricably linked with attitudes of role fulfilment. If role socialisation occurs smoothly because educational objectives are realistic and have been carefully defined, and if the teaching objectives are reinforced by the precept and example of effective role models, the development of desirable attitudes by the student will reinforce the learning process, serve to make learning objectives and activities meaningful and, in turn, generate the drive to acquire the essential knowledge and skills to meet the exacting standards implied by the concept 'quality patient care'. It all depends to what extent the aims, goals and specific objectives of the course provide meaning to the personal and professional life of the student.

Clear objectives are necessary

Only if learning objectives are clearly defined will the student know what she must learn, why she must do so, and when and how she must do it. Such clarity is a debt owed to every student. The hit-and-miss system of clinical teaching used in many nursing schools is a classic example of failure to identify educational objectives and of the lack of interdigitation of the values and scientific content and the lack of moral obligation, both in nurse teaching and to the patient who is a recipient of the student's care. The prejudices against the clear identification of learning objectives in nursing education probably flow from a lack of knowledge and from the rejection of the behaviouristic concepts which dominate the determination of educational objectives to a marked degree. Davies (1976) believes that 'the dogma which has been associated with specific behavioural objectives . . . has often blinded us either to their inherent potential, or to their inbuilt limitations'. He believes that they should not be seen as a universal remedy or panacea for all the ills in contemporary education, but rather as essential tools to guide us and help us to identify the needs of society, patients and learners. Careful identification of objectives leads to clarity in teaching and learning. Richness in teaching and learning need not be restricted for the sake of this essential clarity, and romance in teaching and learning need not be sacrificed for the sake of clarity (Davies 1976: preface). Davies maintains that objectives 'must be put in perspective, and then be handled in a sensitive, creative manner . . . They should be used as a resource for teaching and learning, rather than a set of blinkers or restrainers (Davies 1976: preface). Popham adds to Davies' view by saying that the appropriateness of objectives lies in the clearness, intelligibility, and in the explicitness which are such virtues in teaching (Popham 1972: 32).

Inherent in the need for a clear statement of objectives for quality care is the concept *accurate measurement and evaluation* (or output appraisal), not only of student performance but also of teaching performance. Overshadowing both these components is the question of results. How does all this contribute to quality patient care? Does the health care available to the individual and to society at large meet their needs and expectations? While many of the technical aspects and knowledge comprising nursing can be measured relatively accurately, the complex of activities, attitudes, legal and ethical concepts and applied scientific facts which forms the matrix of nursing care requires an evaluative approach, that is measurement plus judgement formulated in terms of objectives and values. According to Popham, some of our goals and objectives are currently unassessable. Many attitudes and a predisposition to certain actions and standards of accountability will manifest only after some time has elapsed (Popham 1973: 24). This we accept. If we lay a sound foundation we could have reasonable expectations for the future.

Clinical contact is necessary for determining objectives

How can objectives which will contribute to the quality of patient care be developed?

The primary source for the identification of educational objectives for the provision of quality nursing care is the patient himself. Patient health needs and the variables affecting these needs and patient problems in coping with health needs lie at the very heart of a nursing curriculum, and therefore at the heart of educational objectives in the nursing education system. The patient and all the dimensions of his health needs and the problems related thereto are the *raison d'être* for a nursing curriculum.

Teachers of clinical nursing and of the subjects supportive of this cannot determine the educational objectives which will ensure quality care if they are divorced from practice. Such teachers draw only on secondary sources to give form and meaning to their teaching programmes. They rely exclusively on literature and on discussions with their peers to formulate their educational objectives. They are hemmed in by what they imagine are the constraints of the national curriculum. Because the reality of the patient care situation does not leaven their thinking, the educational programme loses its punch and its purpose is misdirected. A tertiary source which is a menace to any educational programme is the bygone experience of the teacher which has had no new inputs from reading, discussion or clinical experience. Although such a teacher may be able to spell out the objectives of a course and its learning experience, the impact is negative because it lacks the reality of the ever-changing, demanding patient care situation.

Society's impact, factors which threaten health, ways of coping with such threats, the human needs of the patient and the potential, aspirations and abilities of nurse and teacher meet at the patient's bedside or his home, school or work situation. His health needs constitute the reason for it all. Yet the teaching of the complex subject, nursing care, is attempted by teachers who stay away from the clinical situation and leave students to cope with the clinical learning situation with the minimum amount of guidance. Without patient involvement by both teacher and nurse, goal-directed educational objectives cannot be determined. In fact, because of misdirection the goal of the newly qualified nurse frequently appears to be 'nursing the administrative procedures', and not the patient. This is described as a widespread phenomenon by many astute nurse observers. Could it possibly be that the absence of scientifically based, clearly defined educational objectives in many of our nursing schools has caused our educational programmes to misfire, with a resultant loss in the qualitative, and in many instances also the quantitative, aspects of nursing care?

Accountability

Accountability in nursing education is of primary importance. Popham (1973: 70) says that the teacher must produce 'evidence regarding the quality of his or her teaching, usually in terms of what happens to the pupils then standing ready to be judged on the basis of the evidence'. The evidence in nursing is quality nursing care. The taxpayer has made the nurse teacher responsible for ensuring that the aims of society for quality nursing care are realised.

Fundamental to accountability are clear aims, goals, objectives and subobjectives in the presentation of the educational programme. The student, the teacher, the assessor of outcomes and society will know exactly where they stand when the nursing curriculum is seen from a broad, total perspective and the objectives are clearly and appropriately defined so as to ensure that the standards set for quality care can be realised. Quality care requires clearly defined standards and accountability, and basic to these are clear-cut, appropriate educational objectives.

References

Burns, R. 1972. *New approaches to behavioral objectives.* 2nd ed. Dubuque: Brown.
Carroll, AD, Duggan, JE & Etchells, R. 1978. *Learning by objectives.* London: Hutchinson.
Clark, DC. 1972. *Using instructional objectives in teaching.* London: Scott Foresman.
Conley, VC. 1973. *Curriculum and instruction in nursing.* Boston: Little Brown.
Davies, I. 1976. *Objectives in curriculum design.* London: McGraw-Hill.
Popham, WJ. 1973. *The use of instructional objectives.* Belmont: Fearon.
Popham, WJ & Baker, EL. 1970. *Establishing instructional goals.* Englewood-Cliffs, NJ: Prentice Hall.

Index